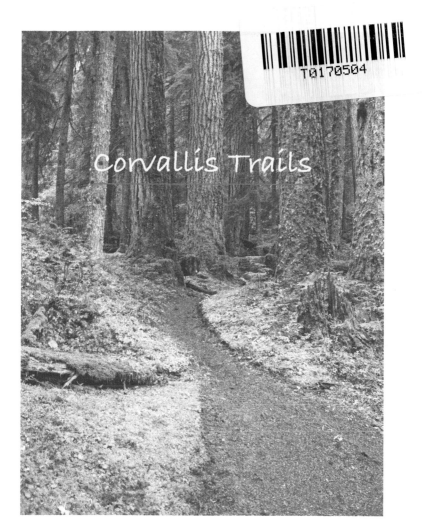

Corvallis Trails

*This guide is dedicated to my hubby, John,
and our kids, Sydney and Lindon,
for the miles of trails we have traveled together.
May there be many more.*

Corvallis Trails

Exploring the Heart of the Valley

Margie C. Powell

Maps
by Tom Bucht

Photographs by
Barry Wulff and Margie C. Powell

Oregon State University Press
Corvallis

Library of Congress Cataloging-in-Publication Data
Powell, Margie C.

Corvallis trails : exploring the heart of the valley / Margie C. Powell ;
maps by Tom Bucht.
p. cm.
Includes index.
ISBN-13: 978-0-87071-099-5 (alk. paper)
ISBN-10: 0-87071-099-0 (alk. paper)
1. Outdoor recreation—Oregon—Corvallis—Guidebooks. 2. Outdoor
recreation—Oregon—Corvallis--Maps. 3. Hiking—Oregon—Corvallis—
Guidebooks. 4. Cycling — Oregon—Corvallis—Guidebooks. 5. Trail
riding--Oregon--Corvallis--Guidebooks. 6. Wilderness areas—Oregon. 7.
Corvallis (Or.)—Description and travel. I. Title.

GV191.42.O7P69 2006
917.95'34—dc22

2006017224

♾ This paper meets the requirements of ANSI/NISO
Z39.48-1992 (Permanence of Paper).

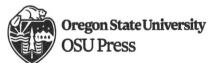

Oregon State University
OSU Press

Oregon State University Press
121 The Valley Library
Corvallis OR 97331
541-737-3166 • fax 541-737-3170
www.osupress.oregonstate.edu

Table of Contents

Acknowledgments

The enthusiastic support of many people made this book possible.

OSU Press editors Mary Braun for planting the seed and seeing it through and Jo Alexander for putting it into book form, despite her broken finger

Barry Wulff for entrusting me with this project and providing his photos

Phil Hays for giving me his "blessing" to write a sequel to his well-used guide

Tom Bucht for his patience and attention to detail in generating the maps and making sure I had it all right

The staff at Benton County Natural Areas and Parks Department, in particular Al Kitzman

The staff at Corvallis Parks and Recreation Department

Trisha Wymore, Recreation Manager for OSU College of Forestry

Traci Merideth, Outdoor Recreation Planner for the Bureau of Land Management

Chantel Jimenez, Recreation Planner for U.S. Fish and Wildlife Service

Photograph credits:
Margie Powell: 28, 41, 45, 48, 56, 63, 69, 78, 81, 98, 100, 122, 124, 126, 132, 137, 144, 147, 152

Barry Wulff: pages i, 5, 10, 12, 13, 17, 20, 22, 30, 36, 50, 51, 53, 59, 65, 71, 76, 85, 86, 89, 102, 105, 109, 111, 113, 129, 141, 151, 154, 162

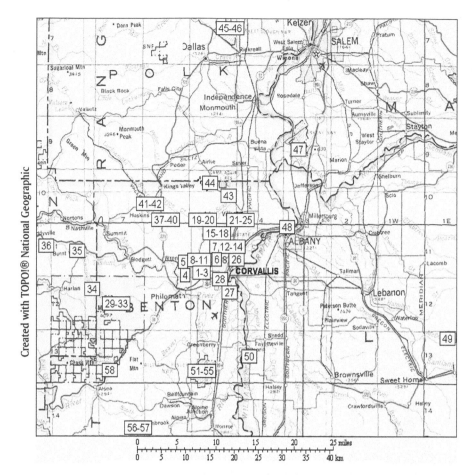

Created with TOPO!® National Geographic

Trail Overview Map

Trail summary chart

Trail number/name	Length	Elevation gain	Diffficulty
Bald Hill Park			
1. Bald Hill Loop	3.1-mi. loop	440 feet	Moderate
2. Mulkey Creek	4.3 mi. round trip	580 feet	Moderate
3. Mulkey Creek to Fitton Green	6.9 mi. round trip	1,170 feet	Moderate to difficult
Fitton Green			
4. Allen Throop Loop	1.2-mi. loop	180 feet	Easy
5. Cardwell Hill Road	5.2 mi. round trip	935 feet	Moderate
Martin Luther King, Jr. Park			
6. MLK Park Loop	1-mi. loop	80 feet	Easy
Chip Ross Park			
7. Chip Ross Park Loop	1.5-mi. loop	310 feet	Easy to moderate
McDonald Forest/Oak Creek			
8. Homestead Trail	1.6-mi. loop	120 feet	Easy
9. Extendo and Uproute trails	4.3-mi. loop	690 feet	Moderate
10. Oak Creek to DimpleHill	7 mi. round trip	1,000 feet	Moderate to difficult
11. Oak Creek to McCulloch Peak	9.3-mi. loop	1,900 feet	Difficult
McDonald Forest/Jackson Creek			
12. Dan's Trail	7.6-mi. round trip	1,400 feet	Moderate
13. Lower Dan's Trail/ Horse Trail Loop	4.8-mi. loop	845 feet	Moderate
14. Upper Dan's Trail/ Horse Trail Loop	8-mi. loop	1,450 feet	Difficult
McDonald Forest/Lewisburg Saddle			
15. Lewisburg Saddle to Dimple Hill	4.8 mi. round trip	545 feet	Moderate
16. Lewisburg Saddle/ Horse Trail Loop	3.2-mi. loop	460 feet	Moderate

Trail number/name	Length	Elevation gain	Diffficulty
17. Vineyard Mountain Loop	6.5-mi. loop	700 feet	Moderate
18. Old Growth Trail	1.6-mi. loop	260 feet	Easy
McDonald Forest/Soap Creek			
19. Baker Creek Trail	0.6 mi. round trip	70 feet	Easy
20. Soap Creek to McCulloch Peak	7.7-mi. loop or 9 mi. round trip	1,600 feet	Difficult
McDonald Forest/Peavy Arboretum			
21. Woodland Trail	0.4-mi. loop	10 feet	Easy
22. Forest Discovery Trail	1.7-mi. loop	270 feet	Easy
23. Intensive Management Trail	1.5-mi. loop	150 feet	Easy
24. Intensive Management/Calloway Creek Loop	3.5-mi. loop	250 feet	Moderate
25. Section 36 Loop and Powderhouse Trail	4-mi. loop	1,030 feet	Moderate
Jackson Frazier Wetland			
26. Bob Frenkel Boardwalk	0.8-mi. loop	insignificant	Easy
Willamette Park			
27. Willamette Park/ KendallNatural Area Loop	2.6-mi. loop	insignificant	Easy
Avery Park			
28. Wildflower Trail/ Avery Park Loop	1.3-mi. loop	insignificant	Easy
Marys Peak			
29. Summit Loop Trail	1.4-mi. loop	385 feet	Easy
30. Meadow Edge Trail	1.8-mi. loop	460 feet	Easy
31. East Ridge/Tie Trail Loop	5.5-mi. loop	1,200 feet	Moderate
32. North Ridge Trail	8.4 mi. round trip	2,165 feet	Difficult
33. North Ridge/ Tie Trail Loop	8.8-mi. loop	1,740 feet	Difficult

Trail number/name	Length	Elevation gain	Diffficulty
Coast Range			
34. Sugarbowl Creek	5 mi. round trip	670 feet	Moderate
35. Strom Boulder Ridge	7.6-mi. loop	1,430 feet	Moderate to difficult
36. Salmon Creek Loop	12-mi. loop	1,900 feet	Moderate to difficult
Beazell Memorial Forest			
37. Bird Loop	1.2-mi. loop	140 feet	Easy
38. South Loop	0.7-mi. loop	150 feet	Easy
39. South Meadow/ Plunkett Creek Loop	2.5-mi. loop	600 feet	Moderate
40. Plunkett Creek Loop	1.8-mi. loop	260 feet	Easy
Fort Hoskins			
41. Recreation Trail	1.6-mi. loop	315 feet	Easy to moderate
42. Interpretive Trail	0.6-mi. loop	85 feet	Easy
Dunn Forest			
43. Soap Creek Loop	6.4-mi. loop	1,150 feet	Moderate
44. Berry Creek Loop	6.3-mi. loop	750 feet	Moderate
Baskett Slough NWR			
45. Baskett Butte	1.4-mi. loop	160 feet	Easy
46. Morgan Lake and Moffitti Marsh Loop Trail	2.5-mi. loop	70 feet	Easy to moderate
Ankeny NWR			
47. Rail Trail Loop	2-mi. loop	15 feet	Easy
Takena Landing			
48. Takena Landing Trail	4 mi.	insignificant	Easy
McDowell Creek Falls			
49. McDowell Creek Falls Loop	1.5-mi. loop	310 feet	Moderate

Trail number/name	Length	Elevation gain	Diffficulty
Snag Boat Bend			
50. Snag Boat Bend Loop	2.1-mi. loop	insignificant	Easy
Finley NWR			
51. Woodpecker Loop	1-mi. loop	130 feet	Easy
52. Mill Hill Trail	3.1-mi. loop	220 feet	Easy
53. Cabell Marsh	2 mi. round trip	50 feet	Easy
54. Beaver/Cattail Pond Loop	2.3-mi. loop	15 feet	Easy
55. Pigeon Butte	3 mi. round trip	285 feet	Easy
Alsea Falls			
56. Alsea River Trail	1-mi. loop	15 feet	Easy
57. Alsea Bike Loop	6-mi. loop	985 feet	Moderate
Clemens Park			
58. Clemens Park Loop	1-mi. loop	15 feet	Easy

INTRODUCTION

Corvallis, Oregon, is a college town pleasantly situated in the Willamette Valley and nestled against the rolling hills of the Coast Range. Indeed, the word "Corvallis" in Latin means "heart of the valley." There are many adjectives that describe our town, including: friendly, welcoming, easy-going, safe, quiet, clean, livable, progressive, healthy, and well educated. Corvallis is rated as one of the most bicycle-friendly towns of its size in the country, because of its very extensive system of bike lanes and paved multi-modal paths. Corvallis also has long been blessed with the foresight of individual citizens and local government leaders who have strived to keep sprawl in check while preserving the natural lands surrounding our community. The result is a system of parks and natural areas, forests and fields, abundant with non-paved trails that are free and accessible to everyone. The purpose of this guide, then, is to direct folks off the pavement and into our little piece of the natural world. The fact that some things in this guide will already be outdated by the time it is published (Fall 2006), and certainly within just a few short years, is really a positive thing. It speaks to the fact that the leaders of our community are continually moving forward with improvements to existing sites and the opening of new lands.

It is common to get stuck in routines, and we all do. This includes where we go to recreate, whether for a daily dose of exercise, or for longer excursions when we have a little more time. My hope is that this guide will present some new ideas for places to explore, whether the reader has lived here for twenty years or two weeks. I hope it proves helpful in deciding where to take or send guests. And finally, I hope that visitors to Corvallis will have access to this guide so that they may discover some of the wonderful spots that our area has to offer.

Outdoor exercise benefits everyone, both physically and mentally. We are fortunate to live in a temperate climate that allows year-round outdoor activity. Spring, summer, and fall easily lure folks outside. When our western Oregon winter arrives, it is often viewed as wet, cold, gray, and unpleasant. It may rain hard sometimes, but often it does not. And compared to real cold, Corvallis is mild. Being outside, moving vigorously in a chilly mist, is refreshing. Our forests and fields can be fascinating in fog and frost and under gray skies; the occasional snow is a treat. Throughout the year there is so much to observe, including the subtle changes from day to day, week to week and season to season. Get out, connect with the natural world, and enjoy yourself. You never know what you may chance upon. And without a doubt, you will have done your body and soul a favor.

How To Use This Book

All the trails in this guide are within an hour's drive of Corvallis. I have divided them into two main sections, Trails Close In and Trails Farther Out. Imagine a circle around the perimeter of Corvallis, within a half-dozen miles of downtown. The Trails Close In section is entirely within this circle. Included are all of Corvallis's city parks with trails, some Benton County lands, and McDonald Forest. These trails are easily reached by most residents and visitors to Corvallis; they are the trails that we can incorporate into our daily lives.

The Trails Farther Out section takes us outside of Corvallis in all directions, but still within an hour's drive. These include some Benton County parks, OSU's Dunn Forest, Marys Peak, four National Wildlife Refuges, two waterfall walks, and some places to explore in the Coast Range. Some of these trails need not be an outing in themselves, but could be included while en route to somewhere else. For example, Snag Boat Bend and Finley Wildlife Refuge are on the way to Eugene; Baskett Slough and Ankeny Wildlife Refuge are on the way to Salem. Clemens Park offers a short walk that is on the way to Waldport and the coast, and everyone passes Takeena Landing just before entering Albany on Highway 20.There are numerous wonderful areas to explore that many are not even aware of.

Within each of these two main sections, the trails are listed in a circle starting at the west and moving around to the north, east, and south. The Overview Map (on page x) showing all the trails by number and the Trail Summary Chart (which begins on page xi) should make it easy to find an appropriate trail based on geography and your tastes. Each trail description includes directions to the trailhead and an information block with the trail length and total elevation gain, difficulty, allowable trail uses, trail surface, and any seasonal closures. A trail identified as "Easy" is generally level and short, a couple of miles or so, with a smooth surface. A trail rated "Moderate" has some elevation gains and losses, is around 5 miles in length, and may have a rougher trail surface. A "Difficult" rating is reserved for trails that climb significantly or are longer than about 7 or 8 miles round trip. All mileages are either for a complete loop or round-trip on an out-and-back trail.

Each trail map has a black flag marking the trailhead; a gray flag on some indicates a secondary trailhead. The described trail is shown with a solid line; an alternate route option or side-trip is shown with a dotted line, as are adjoining trails and roads. Arrows indicate the loop direction that is described. On all maps, north is at the top of the page. An elevation profile is provided if there is elevation change greater than 250 feet. Each park, forest, or natural area is introduced with some background information and a little ecology.

Every effort has been made to assure the accuracy of the information in this book. The author has hiked, run, or biked all the trails and worked with the managing agencies to obtain reliable facts. But neither Oregon State University Press nor the author is responsible for personal injury or other consequences of following directions given in this guide, or for damage to property or violation of the law in connection with the use of this guide.

Corrections and updates are welcome, and will be included in the next edition. Please send them to OSUPress@oregonstate. edu with the subject heading "Corvallis Trails."

Trailhead Parking

There is no fee for parking at any of the trailheads listed in this guide, except for Marys Peak, which requires a Northwest Forest Pass. An annual pass may be purchased locally at the Forest Service office or at sporting good stores and is valid in all Northwest National Forests. This is the way to go if you hike often. Otherwise, a day pass may be purchased for, currently, $5 at the trailhead.

Cars parked at trailheads are sometimes the target of car clouters, otherwise known as opportunistic thieves who bash in windows or jimmy door locks. They are usually after CD players or anything else of value. Do not leave anything valuable in your car, and certainly not in view. Thankfully, this is rarely a problem in our area. Still, take proper precautions and avoid being a victim.

Most trailheads in this area have an adequate, if not official, spot to lock up a bike and bike commuters should feel reasonably comfortable leaving their bike.

Trail Safety and Hazards

Fortunately, the areas covered in this trail guide are fairly benign. The smartest piece of safety advice I could give is to travel with a buddy. Safety in numbers is age-old wisdom. Having said that, I must confess that I often recreate alone, and I generally prefer it that way. I see more, hear more, and think better when I am alone. If you are like me in this regard, at least tell someone where you are going and when you expect to be back. If there is no one available to tell, then leave a note or a message. A dog makes a good companion, especially for females who like to head out on the trails alone. A solitary female should never wear headphones. Stay alert, listen, and look around.

Animals: Cougars, bears, deer, porcupines, skunks, raccoons, coyotes, and bobcats all reside in the forests and fields in and around Corvallis. All will likely see, smell, or hear you coming and will be gone before you ever see them. Cougars are sometimes sighted in McDonald Forest. Read the trailhead notices about recent sightings. If you do see one, don't panic and back away slowly.

Poison Oak: This is the most prolific natural hazard in the Willamette Valley. This innocuous-looking plant carries the oil urushiol on its stems and leaves, causing a skin rash that can range from mildly uncomfortable to severe and scarring. Everyone should learn to recognize and avoid contact with this plant. It is one of the best reasons to stay on the trails in this area.

Poison oak is the most difficult to distinguish in winter with-out its characteristic deeply lobed oak-like leaves. The stems and buds are light brown with a slight velvety appearance. With the arrival of spring, the plant becomes much more recognizable. The opening buds produce very shiny, small, deep red leaves. As spring progresses, the leaves grow and turn green, and are always on a stem in groups of three. In early fall it turns a brilliant red, is quite attractive in the understory, and is a striking vine climbing high up trees. Poison oak often grows in large patches and can be well established in oak forests as well as open areas. It can grow as a low groundcover or as a medium-sized shrubs or tree vine.

When the culprit oil contacts human skin it slowly soaks through the dead outer skin. If you know you have contacted it, wash it off while it is still in this skin layer, if you can. As is frequently the case, exposure is unknown and the oil seeps in to the lower skin level where the irritation begins. A rash or blisters appear from within a few hours to up to a several days after exposure and itching and redness may persist for two or three weeks. Some people are only mildly bothered, while others will require medical attention.

If you know you have been in contact with this plant, the widely accepted treatment is to wash the affected skin areas as

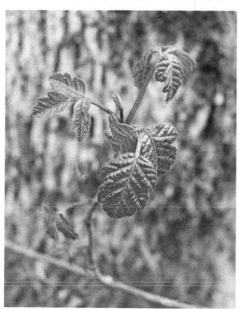

Poison oak in spring

soon as possible with Tecnu, a locally produced skin cleanser. It is wise to keep this product in stock as prompt treatment is the key to successfully avoiding future discomfort. Follow directions on the package. All exposed clothing should be turned inside out and washed thoroughly. If the rash or blisters appear, calamine lotion or a hydrocortisone cream can help relieve the itch in minor cases. If severe lesions form, turning deep red and purple, with obvious infection, see a doctor.

When dogs run through poison oak the oil is deposited on their coat. Many a dog owner receives this "gift" from their canine friend.

Stinging Nettle: Stinging nettle is not nearly the problem in Oregon that poison oak is. While a brush against a nettle will cause an immediate stinging sensation, you will not be in discomfort for the length of time that poison oak continues to torment. A burning or tingling may be accompanied by minor redness and swelling, but the irritation usually lasts from less than an hour to a few days.

This perennial plant appears in spring and is still around in summer. It grows from a few feet to several feet in height and is commonly found in damp, shady areas near streams. Its sharp, serrated leaves are fairly distinct and its tiny, pale green flowers dangle in loose panicles. Its leaves are lined with fine stinging bristles that employ formic acid, the same irritant found in bee and ant stingers. It is an effective defense against animal browsers.

Stinging Insects: Yellow jackets and hornets, which are subfamilies of the wasp, can pose a real hazard in the Willamette Valley. Both of these nest in meadows and forest edges, yellow jackets in the ground and hornets above the ground in tree branches. Hikers may inadvertently step on or brush against a nest. Yellow jackets and hornets are both very protective of their nests, defensive, and will sting repeatedly. Yellow jackets will actually grab on to the innocent perpetrator and sting again and again. In our area they are most abundant in September and, thankfully, all but the young mated females die off quickly with the onset of cold weather.

Most people will suffer only a minor local reaction to the sting: heat, swelling, and itching of the skin around the sting.

Ibuprofen or a sting-relief liquid applied to the skin can ease minor discomfort. The very real hazard is for people who suffer a systemic reaction. Their symptoms include hives, swelling of face, lips, and tongue, and difficulty breathing and swallowing. This life-threatening reaction needs immediate medical attention. People who are known to be highly allergic to insect stings should carry an epi-pen.

Ticks: Lyme disease is the leading tick-borne disease in the U.S. It is primarily a problem in the Northeast and upper Midwest and is less common in the Pacific Northwest. The carrier here is the western black-legged tick, which acquires the culprit bacteria from mice and other animals and then infects humans by burrowing into their skin and passing it into their bloodstream. These ticks live in wooded areas and grasslands.

The ticks are extremely small and easy to overlook. The prudent precaution is to carefully inspect yourself after an outing in brushy areas. Remove a tick by grasping it with tweezers and slowly pulling it out, trying not to break the head off. Squeezing the body will force their fluid under your skin. Save the tick, if possible. If you develop a distinctive red, bulls-eye rash you will want to see a doctor, and bring the tick with you. Later symptoms are similar to the flu.

Giardia: Giardia is a microscopic paramecium that should be suspected in all streams. Drinking untreated water risks getting giardiasis, an illness with symptoms of diarrhea and painful stomach cramps. Avoid this unpleasant ordeal by carrying your own water. Backpackers always use water filters or other forms of water treatment. The days of dipping a cup in a stream are history.

Trees and High Winds: Using the trails during inclement weather can be refreshing. The person who looks wet and pitiful running in the rain may actually enjoy being out in the elements. However, caution is urged in forests in high winds. Soils saturated from heavy rain do not do a very good job anchoring large shallow-rooted trees and strong winds can bring them down. As exhilarating as it may be, windstorms are not the time to be in McDonald Forest, Marys Peak, or other wooded areas.

False Brome: This last hazard is not a danger to the trail user. The danger is to our local environment and we, as recreationists, are part of the ever-growing problem. False brome (*Brachypodium sylvaticum*) is a non-native, exotic grass that is invading habitats in western Oregon at an alarming rate. It is capable of completely dominating both understory and open habitats to the exclusion of most other native species. It currently occupies habitat in the Willamette Valley, coastal forests, and as far south as near the California border. It is prolific in McDonald Forest, at Bald Hill, and in most areas that this trail guide covers. It appears to be tolerant of fire, and mowing and burning as methods of control are mostly ineffective. Herbicide application may be effective in small areas.

False Brome can be distinguished from other grasses by its fountain-like habit, broad leaves, hairy leaf margins and lower stems, and its long-lasting bright green color. Its flower spikes droop noticeably. Resource management agencies are trying to get a handle on this ecological nightmare. They are trying to keep the grasses cut back from the trail edges so trail users don't brush against them. They are employing methods for cleaning their equipment so as not to transport the seeds to other locations. We, as recreationists, must do our part to help control the spread. First, learn to recognize it. False brome seeds readily cling to our shoes, clothing, backpacks, bicycles, car tires, and to our pets. Make every effort to stay on trails and roads to minimize exposure to the seeds. Before leaving the trailhead, look for and brush off the innocent-looking seeds that have clung to you, your gear or your dog.

Good Trail Manners

Many folks share our trails and in a variety of uses. These trails belong to all of us. Let us not forget our good manners, as it reflects on our community as a whole.

• Do not cut switchbacks or take shortcuts. It damages the resource, causes erosion problems, and looks tacky.

• Do not pick wildflowers. Leave them for those who follow to enjoy.

• Litter is blessedly scarce on our trails but if you do see some, be a good steward and take it out.

• Dogs are great trail companions where allowed. Leave an aggressive dog at home, however. Keep your dog on a leash or within voice command. Not everyone wants to be greeted and sniffed by even the friendliest of pooches. Always control your dog around bikers and horses; they do not know your dog's temperament.

• The rule of thumb for trail right-of-way is this: Hikers, runners, and bikers should yield to horses. Try to step off the trail on the downhill side to let horses pass. Bikers should yield to hikers and runners; however, my observation is that hikers and runners instinctively yield to bikers.

• Respect private property where public trails and roads pass through or skirt along the edge.

• Look at trailhead information kiosks. In addition to their general information, there may be notices of things that the managing agency wants you to be aware of.

• Heed seasonal closure signs. They are generally for wet trail conditions or wildlife sanctuary. The information block with each trail description in this guide includes seasonal closures, but there may be additional temporary closures.

How to Get Involved

Groups to Recreate With: If you enjoy the camaraderie of recreating with like-minded folks there are some local organizations that would welcome your company. These groups generally send out calendars of upcoming outings and carpool from preset meeting places. They are:

    Marys Peak Group of the Sierra Club:
        www.oregon.sierraclub.org/groups/marys_peak
    Greenbelt Land Trust: www.greenbeltlandtrust.
        org or send email for information to: info@
        greenbeltlandtrust.org or call: 541-752-9609
    The Audubon Society: www.audubon.corvallis.or.us
    Mid-Valley Bicycle club www.peak.org/-mvbc
    Oregon Equestrian Trails www.oregonequestriantrails.org

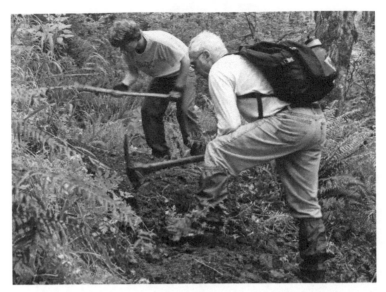

Groups That Help Develop and Maintain Trails: The trails in this area cannot possibly be built and maintained by paid staff alone. They rely on and hugely appreciate volunteer help. It is fun and extremely rewarding to volunteer on trails. There are two organizations that regularly help the City of Corvallis, Benton County, the U.S. Forest Service, the Bureau of Land Management, and the U.S. Fish and Wildlife Service. You do not have to be a member of these groups to help out. They are:

> Marys Peak Group of the Sierra Club:
> > www.oregon.sierraclub.org/groups/marys_peak
> Greenbelt Land Trust: www.greenbeltlandtrust.
> > org or send email for information to: info@
> > greenbeltlandtrust.org or call: 541-752-9609
> To volunteer on the trails on McDonald Forest or to
> > become a Volunteer Trail Patroller: www.cof.orst.edu/
> > cf/recreation/volunteer_info.php or call: 541-737-6703

For More Information

The information block for each trail identifies the resource managing agency. For additional information go to their website or call their office.

Corvallis Parks and Recreation www.ci.corvallis.or.us
541-766-6918
Benton County Natural Areas and Parks www.co.benton.
or.us 541-766-6871
OSU College of Forestry www.cof.edu/resfor 541-737-
4452 (office) or 541-737-4434 (recorded info)
Siuslaw National Forest www.fs.fed.us/r6/siuslaw 541-
750-7000
Bureau of Land Management www.or.blm.gov/salem
503-375-5646
Willamette Valley National Wildlife Refuge Complex
www.willamettevalley.fws.gov 541-757-7236
Linn County Parks www.co.linn.or.us/parks 541-967-
3917

Going Beyond the Area Covered in this Guide

There are many guide books available for recreating in Oregon,
hiking in particular. The ones below, as well as those going
beyond Oregon, can be purchased at our local bookstores or
borrowed from the Corvallis-Benton County Public Library.
100 Hikes in the Central Oregon Cascades, third edition,
by William L. Sullivan. Navillus Press.
100 Hikes in Southern Oregon, second edition, by
William L. Sullivan. Navillus Press.
100 Hikes in Northwest Oregon, second edition, by
William L. Sullivan. Navillus Press
100 Hikes on the Oregon Coast and Coast Range, second
edition, by William L. Sullivan. Navillus Press.
*Best Hikes with Children in Western and Central
Oregon*, second edition, by Bonnie Henderson. The
Mountaineers Books.
120 Hikes on the Oregon Coast, second edition, by
Bonnie Henderson. The Mountaineers Books.
Oregon's Best Wildflower Hikes, Northwest Region, by
George Wuerthner. Westcliff Publishers.
Best Hikes with Dogs, Oregon, by Ellen Morris Bishop.
The Mountaineers Books.

Bald Hill Park

Bald Hill Park, west of the Benton County Fairgrounds, is perhaps Corvallis's most successful trail-development system. It is a close-in natural park of 284 acres that residents love and use regularly. Trail users range from trail runners and joggers, birdwatchers, dog and fitness walkers, bike commuters and equestrians, to families with strollers, roller skaters, and youngsters learning to ride a bike. Bald Hill offers 2.5 miles of rolling asphalt and close to 7 miles of dirt and gravel trails with countless ways to create loops of any distance. During the winter months the trails out in the open can help lift one's spirit. Those tucked in the woods have their own appeal in cold winter fog and provide a shady respite in the heat of the summer. In spring and fall the park is lovely everywhere. The trails pass through oak woodlands and grasslands, riparian areas, active grain farming and the free-range beef and lamb farms owned by Bald Hill Farms, LCC. The park's name comes from the prominent hill, which used to be referred to as Old Baldy. Oak woodlands and Douglas firs have crept up the sides

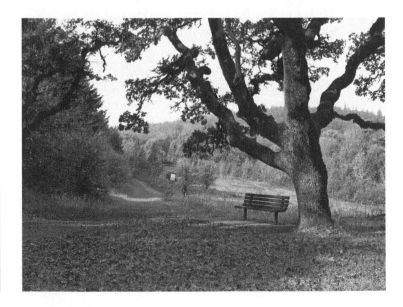

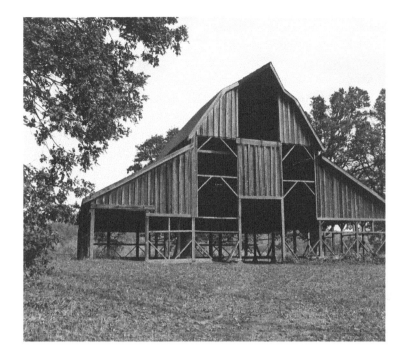

and now only the west side is bald. The view to the south and west from the top is satisfying. The City of Corvallis manages the park. The Nature Conservancy and the Greenbelt Land Trust have partnered with the City to restore the oak savanna and native grass prairie through removal of invasive nonnative species. Much of the trail maintenance is done by volunteers.

Bald Hill Park's history is worth mentioning, as it truly showcases the community's efforts to provide areas for recreation. In the late 1970s OSU allowed for a public easement to connect the west end of campus with the Fairgrounds. In 1985 the Coon family donated 60 acres to the City of Corvallis and it was named Bald Hill Park. Their home site's barn still stands and has become a treasured landmark. In the 1990s, the City of Corvallis and Benton County collaborated with an adjacent landowner, Jack Brandis, to allow a public easement connecting the Fairgrounds to the park. This is the multimodal paved path now named the Midge Cramer Memorial Path, honoring a long-time bicycle advocate for our area. During this same time the City and County together developed the trail system within the park and also worked with landowner Andrew Martin to extend the trail to the west end of his property along Mulkey Creek. In 2001 Martin donated an easement along Oak Creek to Benton County Natural Areas and Parks Department, which developed the trail link with Mulkey Creek. In 2003 an easement was provided by Greg Hammerstad to connect Mulkey Creek with Fitton Green to the west (see page 19). The County and the Marys Peak Group of the Sierra Club built this link, which takes folks to Fitton Green via Wynoochee and Panorama Dr. We are fortunate to have access to this extensive area and should always be respectful of the private properties these trails pass through.

To get there: Parking and access are available at three entrances. One parking area is on the south side of Oak Creek Rd., 0.75 mile west from the Harrison Blvd./53rd St./Walnut Blvd./Oak Creek Rd. junction. Another small lot is on the north side of Reservoir Rd., 1 mile west of 53rd St. Unlimited parking exists at the west end of the Fairgrounds parking lot.

Trail 1. Bald Hill Loop Trail

Length: 3.1-mile loop • Elevation gain: 440 feet
Difficulty: Moderate •Trail uses: Foot, bike, horse
Trail surface: Paved, gravel, packed earth (muddy in
  rainy weather)
Seasonal closures: From barn to top on southeast side
  closed to bikes and horses 10/31 to 4/15
Managing agency: City of Corvallis
Other information: Dog off-leash area. Stay on the
  trails; poison oak is thick in the oak woodlands.

There are several ways to create loops at Bald Hill and everyone has their favorites. The following describes a loop that begins and ends at the Oak Creek parking area.

Follow the paved path south for 0.4 miles. Turn right up the hill to the barn. (The barn is 1.2 miles from the Reservoir Road entrance and 1.1 miles from the Fairgrounds entrance, if you are coming in from those entrances.) Just below the barn, pass an old access road on the left designated for horse use; it is not the best choice for those on foot. Turn left across from the barn and head southwest, immediately entering dense oak woods. Keep an eye out for a small grove of enormous Madrone trees that you will pass under. Their smooth, reddish brown, flaky bark stands in contrast to the oaks, maples, and invading Douglas-firs. At 0.8 miles pass the Mardi Keltner Interpretive Trail branching off to the right. This short, foot-travel-only interpretive trail playfully curves and undulates and reconnects back with the loop trail on the west side. The Loop Trail continues straight, crosses the horse route and curves up the east and south sides of Bald Hill. On the left, pass a switchbacking connector trail coming up from the paved path near the Reservoir Road entrance. Proceeding on up, some views to the south begin to emerge. At 1.4 miles there is a bench and a fine spot to look around. The actual top of "Old Baldy" is about 100 yards further up the path to the east. There is a bench there as well, and a good spot for a picnic. Continuing around Bald Hill, the trail winds down through oak woodlands. At 1.8 miles the west end of the Mardi Keltner trail joins in from the right. The loop trail turns east through open

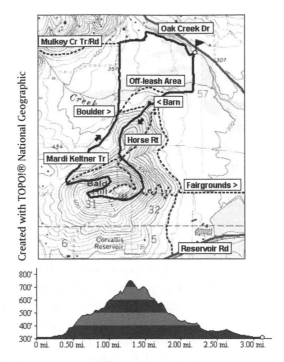

oak prairie. At the next junction, identified by an appreciation boulder to landowner Andrew Martin, turn left. (Straight ahead returns you to the barn; the trail in the middle returns you to the paved path below the barn through a designated dog off-leash area). This level trail heads north for 0.3 miles with bridge crossings over several small branches of Mulkey Creek. Pass between grazing fields to connect to the Mulkey Creek trail/road. Turn right and follow the road almost to Oak Creek Dr. Turn right again and follow the trail back along Oak Creek to the parking area.

Trail 2. Mulkey Creek Trail

Length: 4.3 miles round trip • Elevation gain: 580 feet
Difficulty: Moderate • Trail uses: Foot, bike, horse
Trail surface: Gravel, packed earth (top half muddy
   during rainy season)
Seasonal closures: Closed above bridge at mile 1.3 to
   bikes and horses 10/31 to 4/15
Managing agency: Benton County

From the trailhead on Oak Creek Dr., cross the bridge and immediately turn right, heading west. The gravel path passes through Bald Hill Farms, paralleling Oak Creek Dr. and Oak Creek itself. Killdeer are often seen swooping through the fields and Blue Herons are not uncommon. Following trail signs continue west and gradually uphill along a gravel road through sheep and cattle farming fields and a couple home sites. The actual trail begins at the end of the road, immediately entering the narrow shady corridor of Mulkey Creek, with steep fern-covered hillsides and dense oak, maple, and Douglas-fir woods. In spring the wildflowers burst into bloom, including beautiful large white and pink trillium lilies, bleeding hearts, and many more. At 1.2 miles from the parking area, the trail to Fitton Green leaves to the right. Continue west (left) and cross Mulkey Creek on a sturdy footbridge. The trail now switchbacks up

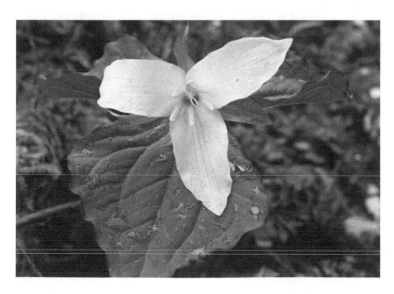

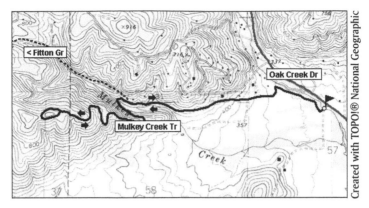

Created with TOPO!® National Geographic

through a steep wooded hillside. The shady environment has encased the trees in moss, creating beautiful fern gardens high in the branches. Further up, the forest opens giving a view to the south of Bald Hill Park. The bench here was a gift of appreciation to Denise Nervik for her tireless contributions to trail development and maintenance in Benton County. The trail continues to climb, more gradually, through attractive open woods. For the time being, the trail loops back on itself at the west end of Andrew Martin's property. Retrace your steps back to the trailhead.

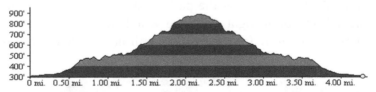

Created with TOPO!® National Geographic

Trail 3. Mulkey Creek to Fitton Green

Length: 6.9 miles round trip • **Elevation gain**: 1,170 feet
Difficulty: Moderate to difficult • **Trail uses**: Foot,
bike, horse
Trail surface: Gravel
Seasonal closures: Fitton Green closed to bikes and
horses 10/31 to 4/15
Managing agency: Benton County

At the time of this printing, the only way to reach Fitton
Green from Bald Hill is to start at the trailhead on Oak Creek
Dr.Turn right immediately after crossing the bridge and follow
the Mulkey Creek Trail directions to the junction at mile 1.2;
turn right (the Mulkey Creek Trail continues to the left). Follow
this short spur trail, leaving the cool corridor of Mulkey Creek
for wide, graveled Wynoochee Dr. Proceed west (left) on
Wynoochee for 0.9 miles, climbing steadily to the junction with
Panorama Dr. Turn left and continue another 0.6 miles up past
homes nestled into the forest. The road tops out and gently
drops past the last home and into Fitton Green Natural Area.
Follow the grassy park road for 100 yards, turn left, and loop
around Fitton Green clockwise. (Refer to the Fitton Green trail
description.) Retrace your steps back down to the parking lot.

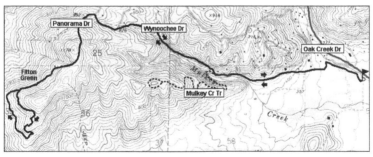

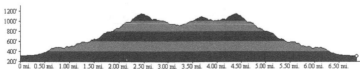

Created with TOPO!® National Geographic

Fitton Green Natural Area

Fitton Green Natural Area, formerly referred to as Open Space Park, lies to the west of Bald Hill Park. This 308-acre property overlooks the valleys of the Marys and Willamette rivers, and the town of Philomath. The views of Marys Peak and the Coast Range are terrific. The old Cardwell Hill Road passes through the northern section of the property. The park's significance to our area dates to 1988. This is when Charles and Elsie Ross created and endowed the Greens Trust Fund to begin purchasing open space parcels to surround our communities. They were guided by the philosophy of retaining "permanently some of the green fields and wooded hills where we can see them daily and reach them easily ..." (Charles Ross, 1999). This led to Benton County's purchase of the first 85 acres and also gave birth to the Greenbelt Land Trust. In 1995 and 1998 the Greenbelt purchased and donated an additional 223 acres. The Greenbelt Land Trust continues working with Benton County and the City of Corvallis to acquire critical open space lands, which can then be made accessible to the public. The name Fitton was chosen because it was Elsie Ross's name before she married. Fitton Green formally opened in 2004.

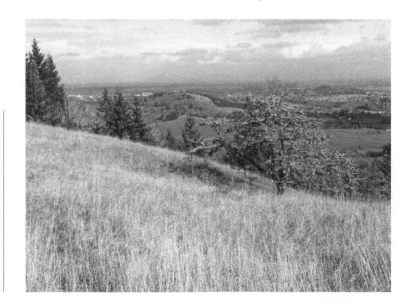

The top of Fitton Green is a natural area with oak groves and grasslands, but it hasn't always been this way. Upland prairie like this is an endangered ecosystem in the Northwest. Native Americans kept the land cleared with frequent burnings. As European settlers moved in, open woodlands were mostly converted to agriculture or replaced by closed-canopy forest. Grazing and two cycles of intensive logging occurred on the Fitton Green site prior to County ownership. Time and continued habitat restoration will further the healing of this knoll. A rare butterfly, the Taylor's Checkerspot, which is appropriately OSU orange and black, thrives near Fitton Green and the hope is that eventually the species will populate Fitton Green as well. Lower in the park the vegetation is mixed Douglas-fir and hardwood forest, and a riparian forest exists along the fish-bearing stream parallel to Cardwell Hill Road.

There is a 1.2-mile loop trail through the open meadow at the top and a 1-mile trail from the top down to Cardwell Hill Road.

To get there: Parking and access are available at three locations. Proceed west on Oak Creek Dr. from the Harrison Blvd./ 53rd St. junction 2 miles, and continue straight onto Cardwell Hill Dr. for 0.7 miles. Where Cardwell Hill Dr. turns to gravel, continue straight and proceed steeply uphill to the Cardwell Hill East trailhead parking.

For a second access, turn left on Chinook Dr. from Cardwell Hill Dr. At the top of the hill at the T junction at 0.5 miles, turn right on Chaparral Dr. This becomes Panorama Dr. Follow brown county park signs for 1.5 miles to the park entrance and trailhead parking.

From the community of Wren, the Cardwell Hill West trailhead is at the gated end of Cardwell Hill Dr., 1.7 miles east from Kings Valley Hwy. 223.

From Bald Hill Park, foot, bicycle, and horse access is by following the Mulkey Creek trail 1.2 miles to the signed junction with the link trail to Wynooche Dr. Turn left and follow Wynooche Dr. 0.9 miles; turn left on Panorama Dr., and continue 0.6 miles to the park entrance.

Trail 4. The Allen Throop Loop at Fitton Green

Length: 1.2-mile loop • Elevation gain: 180 feet
Difficulty: Easy • Trail uses: Foot, bike, horse
Trail surface: Gravel, grassy road
Seasonal closures: Closed to bikes and horses 10/31 to
4/15
Managing agency: Benton County

An outing to Fitton Green from the trailhead at the end of Panorama Dr. is a rare opportunity to enjoy a splendid hilltop vista and a walk or a picnic without a long uphill trudge to get there. Of course the view is all the more satisfying if you have come up either from Bald Hill or Cardwell Hill on your own set of lungs, but starting from this trailhead is a real treat.

This trail system is dedicated to Allen Throop, a man who devoted much of his life to preserving open spaces and creating trails in the Corvallis area. His work with the Greenbelt Land Trust was instrumental in acquiring Fitton Green and other unique parcels of land. He passed away in 2004 as this trail was being constructed.

From the kiosk, head southwest on an old and wide, grassy road. At the first junction veer left and proceed slightly uphill to the high point of the park and a panoramic view. Behind you looms a large home that you may have seen from other vantage spots in the area. The irregular shape of the Fitton Green property has a notch cut out that is privately owned.

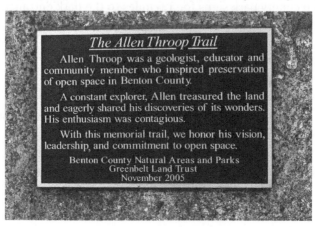

The Allen Throop Trail

Allen Throop was a geologist, educator and community member who inspired preservation of open space in Benton County.

A constant explorer, Allen treasured the land and eagerly shared his discoveries of its wonders. His enthusiasm was contagious.

With this memorial trail, we honor his vision, leadership, and commitment to open space.

Benton County Natural Areas and Parks
Greenbelt Land Trust
November 2005

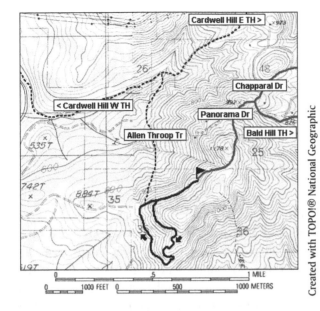

Please respect this boundary. After taking in the great view, head south down the gravel trail, which gently switchbacks through the open meadow. The short trail then empties onto an old haul road and heads back up the hill to the trailhead.

For a longer outing turn left at the signed junction. Follow the Allen Throop Trail, an old grassy road that drops down one mile through mixed forest. It is muddy in places during the wet months. Intersect the old Cardwell Hill Rd. about half way along its length between the two gated east and west trailheads. To make the outing a little longer yet, turn left and follow the road to the Marys River before turning around. Return up the old road back to the main Fitton Green loop. Turn left and continue back up to the parking area and kiosk.

Trail 5. Cardwell Hill Road

Length: 5.2 miles round trip • **Elevation gain:** 935 feet
Difficulty: Moderate • **Trail uses:** Foot, bike, horse
Trail surface: Graveled and grassy road, muddy in
    places in rainy weather
Seasonal closures: Open year round
Managing agency: Benton County

A trek along the old Cardwell Hill Rd. offers a great opportunity for some honest exercise. Though the trail is not too long, there is a steep climb in both directions. Formerly called County Road 10, this road was built in 1855 to connect Wren with Corvallis. William Cardwell lived along the road and eventually the road came to bear his name. Along with local "traffic" the road carried supplies and troops from the riverfront of Corvallis to Fort Hoskins in Kings Valley from 1856 to 1865. In the early 1900s the road was still very much a part of the County road system. It has now long since been closed to vehicles, but is still a dedicated public right-of-way. The road climbs steeply out of the Oak Creek drainage and then winds down into and along the Marys River drainage. It can be muddy in the wet months but the road surface is hugely improved since it became a formal access to Fitton Green.

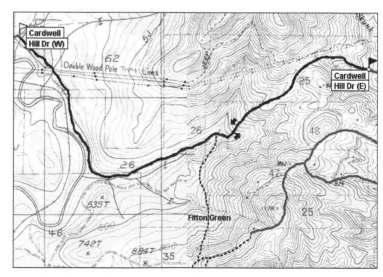

Created with TOPO!® National Geographic

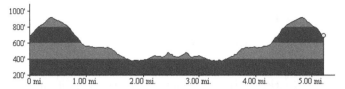

Created with TOPO!® National Geographic

The trail description starts at the Cardwell Hill East trailhead. From the information kiosk, head west. Decades of erosion and poor drainage have created a road bed that now sits in a trough up to 6 feet deep in places. This has given it a magical, hobbit-like feeling, as ferns, mosses, and other plants have grown along the shady walls. The uphill is steady for the first 0.3 miles to the high point at 900 feet elevation. The south side of the trail is mostly Douglas-fir woods, while the north side is heavily cut, private forest lands. From the top the view back is of the Oak Creek drainage and Dimple Hill in McDonald Forest. Just down the other side of the summit, keep a lookout on the left for an enormous "wolf tree." This magnificent multi-trunked Douglas-fir is nothing like all the other straight-standing younger Douglas-fir trees and speaks of an origin on an open ridge top. These legacy trees are valuable for wildlife and are not often seen.

The road now winds down through mixed Douglas-fir and hardwood forest. You will come to a junction with the 1-mile Allen Throop Trail up to Fitton Green. Continue west as the road gently descends in a broadening valley. As the road makes a sharp curve to the north, it now follows along the Marys River, serenely making its way to Corvallis and the Willamette River. The railroad to Toledo crosses the river on a trestle here and turns to the west. The trail then passes through a self-closing gate and crosses private grazing lands. The Cardwell Hill West trailhead is just outside a second gate. This would be the logical turn-around spot.

Dr Martin Luther King Jr. Park
(formerly Walnut Park)

Dr. Martin Luther King Jr. Park is a 30-acre community park on the northwest side of Corvallis. It was acquired into the City's park system as Walnut Park in 1965. It was renamed Dr. Martin Luther King Jr. Park in 2005. There is a semi-enclosed barn on the north side of the park that can be rented for parties and reunions. Nearby are a children's play area and picnic tables, as well as ball fields and a large grass field along Walnut Blvd. that is popular with Frisbee throwers. From the graveled parking area off Walnut Blvd. a paved path runs 0.5 mile northwest through the park and connects with Ponderosa Ave. This path is well used by residents living at both ends as it passes through open wetlands alive with birds, rabbits, deer, and elusive coyote. For a longer walk, many folks starting here often continue up through the quiet, hilly, and shady neighborhood of Skyline and loop back down to the park. Large stands of camas grow in this park. Rising above blankets of yellow violets, it makes a nice display in April and May. Native Americans relied on this bulb for food and while most of it in the Willamette Valley has long since been plowed under, it can easily be found here. By mid-summer the south-facing hill is covered with non-native but quite pretty Queen Ann's lace and the blackberry picking is exceptionally good.

To get there: From Walnut Blvd. heading west, the park is on the right as the road swings south, to become 53rd St. Heading north on 53rd St. from the Fairgrounds, the park is on the left, 1.4 miles from the Oak Creek Rd./Harrison Blvd./53rd St./ Walnut Blvd. intersection.

Trail 6. MLK Park Loop Trail

Length: 1-mile loop • **Elevation gain:** 80 feet
Difficulty: Easy • **Trail uses:** Foot
Trail surface: Gravel, packed earth
Seasonal closures: Open year round
Managing agency: City of Corvallis
Other information: Dog off-leash area

The loop trail starts at the drinking fountain, portable restroom, and dog-duty station area where the paved path begins. Proceed south along the edge of the long grassy field. A small stream with an abundance of cattails separates you from the ball fields. At the south end of the park a bridge will take you over the stream and through a short but pleasant riparian area into an open meadow. A fabulously landscaped private estate complete with a lavender farm lies to the south in this former wetland. Though dogs are permitted off leash in this area of the park, it is an enjoyable stroll for non-dog owners as well. As the trail climbs slightly and turns north, informal trails head further west into the adjacent neighborhood and woods. They can be fun for children to explore and, in early spring, there is a wonderful spread of pink calypso orchids (commonly called fairy slippers) that I would encourage any fan of these special flowers to seek out. Be aware of poison oak, however. The gravel trail continues along the western edge of the park, utilizing a short span of volunteer-built boardwalk, to protect

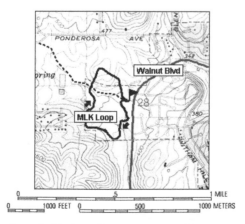

Created with TOPO!® National Geographic

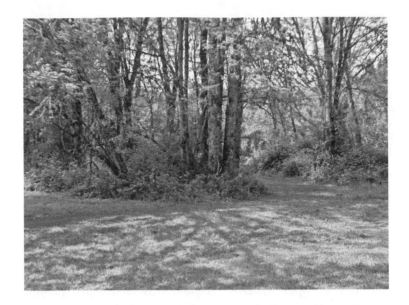

the soggy soil. Cross another small stream on a bridge and then cross the paved path and continue up the open slope. The view from the top of the surrounding hillsides, neighborhoods, and the Cascades to the east is worth the increase in heart rate. Turn east and follow the path down to the barn and the start of the loop. Runners have been known to do multiple loops as part of their training.

Chip Ross Park/
Timberhill Open Space

There is a certain pleasure to be derived from climbing up above a town, whether one is a resident or a visitor, and looking down upon it, picking out landmarks, seeing where it is situated and how it is laid out. Chip Ross Park and Timberhill Open Space offer an easily accessible place to do just that. Dimple Hill, further to the west, has an even finer view but is not as easily reached. This area also serves as an entry to the many roads and trails of McDonald Forest.

Chip Ross Park, comprising 126 hilltop acres of oak savannah, is on the northern edge of Corvallis above the Timberhill area. It overlooks Corvallis and the Willamette Valley, with views of the Cascades and Coast Range. This property was the first one donated into the City's Open Space Plan in 1979. Charles and Elsie Ross gave this land, which had been sold to them for this purpose by Dan and Dorothy Petroquin, to Corvallis in honor of their son, Charles (Chip) Fitton Ross. Harold Nelson and others donated land to enlarge the park. The Greenbelt Land Trust and the Corvallis Open Space Commission were instrumental in securing passage of the 2000 Open Space Bond Measure, which added an additional 47 acres to the south side of the park. Several rocks and benches memorialize former citizens. As development continues to push up the hills on the north side of Corvallis, it is easy to appreciate these parcels of land that have been set aside for all to enjoy.

To get there: There are several ways to access Chip Ross Park and Timberhill Open Space. The official Chip Ross Park trailhead is at the end of Lester Ave. From Walnut Blvd., take Highland Dr. north for 0.9 miles. Turn left on Lester Ave. The trailhead is in 0.7 miles at the end of the road; here you will find an information kiosk, picnic tables, and a portable rest room. The loop trail starts and finishes here.

Secondary trail access is from the top of 29th St. From Walnut Blvd., head north for 1 mile to the information kiosk and roadside parking. This access is through Timberhill Open Space. Take the right fork heading east from the trailhead for

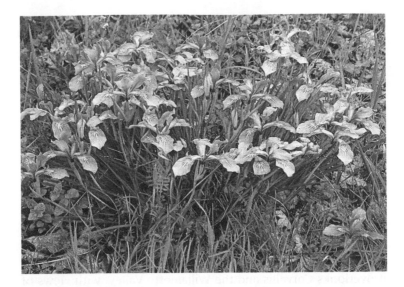

0.4 miles climbing the hill to intersect Chip Ross Park Loop on the lower trail. Turn right and make the loop from here. The left fork from the top of 29th St. accesses McDonald Forest and Dan's Trail (trail 12).

For an even longer uphill walk or run, start on the paved path just east of Timberhill Athletic Club. The pavement ends promptly and an informal and often muddy track on the developer's property takes the most direct route and that is straight up. Intersect the Chip Ross Park Loop on the lower trail. As development continues in this area, this access will change.

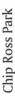

Trail 7. Chip Ross Park Loop

Length: 1.5-mile loop • **Elevation gain:** 310 feet
Difficulty: Easy to moderate • **Trail uses:** Foot, bike, horse
Trail surface: Packed earth, some gravel. Very muddy in rainy weather
Seasonal closures: Closed to bikes and horses 11/1 to 4/15
Managing agency: City of Corvallis
Other information: The poison oak off the trail is thick

From the official trailhead on Lester Ave., proceed north on the easternmost trail (the one on the right) and make the loop counterclockwise. The trail starts at a gentle climb, with dense oak woods on the left and an open field on the right. As you wrap around to the west you look into Crescent Valley. The trail climbs more steeply but at 0.5 mile levels off in a broad open oak prairie. Enjoy far-ranging views as you continue west along the ridge. A couple of user-made tracks drop straight down the hill. These informal trails are the quickest way up or down the hill, but are not particularly pleasant in either

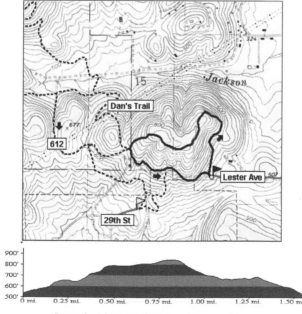

Created with TOPO!® National Geographic

direction and using them continues to damage the resource. At the last bench, the trail forks; both drop steeply and come together at the bottom. The left fork is a little better. Where they come together, there is a four-way junction. Turn left and loop back on the lower trail to the Lester Ave. trailhead or the Timberhill Open Space access.

An enjoyable loop of another 1.5 miles, including the first section of Dan's Trail, can be added. At the previous four-way junction, which is the start of Dan's Trail (see trail 12), continue straight ahead. After a gradual descent into the Jackson Creek basin, veer left at the next junction in 0.59 miles and then intersect Rd. 612 in another 0.24 miles. Leave Dan's Trail here, turning left on Rd 612. Climb to the ridge, and follow this road as it loops back to the east. Just before the water tank, veer left and you will be back at the four-way junction in Chip Ross Park. Turn right and follow the lower trail to your starting point.

McDonald Forest: Introduction

McDonald Forest covers 7,250 acres in the hilly country north and northwest of Corvallis. Further north, another 4,000 acres comprise the Dunn Forest (see page 119). McDonald-Dunn is public land managed by OSU College of Forestry and its primary goal is to enhance forest research, teaching, and demonstration, as well as being a principal financial asset of the college. At any one time there are usually forty to eighty research projects under way in the forest and more than forty university classes receive instruction in the forest each year.

Add in more than 150,000 recreational visits each year from hikers, runners, mountain bikers, and equestrians and you can appreciate an additional goal of the college, which is to provide safe, quality recreation for the very recreation-oriented community of Corvallis. While researchers do experience some vandalism at their project sites, most forest recreation visitors pass benignly through. OSU recognizes the opportunity to educate the public on forest management practices and continues to invest in developing and maintaining a high-quality trail system. There are currently 19 miles of trails open to foot travel year-round with bicycles and horses allowed on some trails during the dry season. In addition there are 64 miles of forest roads open to foot, bicycle, and horse travel year round, with the exception of posted, temporary closures.

For thousands of years Naive Americans lived in these hills. Their purposeful and regular burning produced an open landscape which provided important subsistence plants and animals. As elsewhere in the Willamette Valley, epidemics and the arrival of Euro-American explorers decimated the tribes in the early 1800's. Homesteaders settled in and logging and agriculture gradually changed the valley's ecosystem. The McDonald portion of the forest was acquired by gifts and purchases from 1925 to 1962. Mary McDonald was a primary benefactress, donating land and money to the OSU College of Forestry. Deans George Peavy and Paul Dunn, and Professor T. J. Starker were also instrumental in acquiring forest lands for the college.

McDonald Forest is dominated by Douglas-fir of various ages. In lesser numbers are grand firs, western red cedars, big leaf maples, and white oaks. A large number of plant species comprise the understory, including an abundance of spring wildflowers. More than a hundred plant species in the forest are non-native and some are aggressive invaders. The most notable is False-brome (*Brachypodium sylvaticum*). This exotic, perennial grass is rapidly invading McDonald Forest and elsewhere in the Corvallis area. Forest recreation users contribute to its spread. To become more familiar with this nightmare plant, please read more about it in the introduction to this guide.

Deer and small mammals such as chipmunks and squirrels are commonly observed here, while mountain lions, bobcats, black bears, and coyotes are present but infrequently seen.

For the forest recreational visitor to better understand why their recreational outings sometimes take them through unsightly new clear-cuts and other times through diverse and undisturbed forest, a brief explanation of OSU College of Forestry's four themes of management may be helpful. Each theme offers a distinct and different set of forest values and uses. Theme 1 areas maximize yield of Douglas-fir on short rotations, i.e., they are tree plantations. This theme is dominant in the Dunn Forest and the Soap Creek area of McDonald Forest. Theme 2 optimizes yield of high-quality Douglas-fir, but on longer rotations. Theme 2 comprises most of the rest of the Dunn Forest, the McCulloch Peak area, and much of the land east of the Lewisburg Saddle. Theme 3 retains tree cover for a more visually pleasing harvesting process and comprises much of the forest viewed from Corvallis. Theme 4 provides diverse forest habitats. Most of Oak Creek, Jackson Creek, the west side of Lewisburg Saddle, and Peavy Arboretum are managed in this way and, hence, that is where the best recreation opportunities occur. In addition, there are many small pockets of old-growth reserve scattered throughout.

All of McDonald Forest is managed by the OSU College of Forestry. Their rules are as follows: Remain on official trails and roads. Recreation is allowed from dawn to dusk. No overnight camping is allowed. Fire building, smoking, and consuming alcohol are not allowed. No shooting is allowed except during the seasonal hunt with an OSU seasonal access permit. Plants may not be cut, collected, picked, or removed. Motor vehicles are not allowed past gates; however recreational users on forest roads should be alert for occasional authorized vehicles. Observe area, trail, and road closures. Some trails are open year round to bikes and horses; others are open to these uses only from April 15 to October 31. Do not ride on muddy trails. If trails are extraordinarily wet late into the spring, closures may be extended. Leave research projects undisturbed. Read trailhead notices for current information, closures, etc. And lastly, hikers, runners, and bicyclists yield to horses; bicyclists yield to hikers and runners. If you are interested in volunteering for trail maintenance or to join the Volunteer Trail Patrol, call 737-6703.

I have divided the McDonald Forest trail descriptions into five geographic areas in order, generally, from west to east: Oak Creek area, Jackson Creek area, Lewisburg Saddle area, Soap Creek area, and Peavy Arboretum. A brief introduction to each area and access directions precedes the trail descriptions. To ease trailhead parking congestion, consider biking to the trailhead whenever possible. While some entry points may seem busy, especially on weekends, the forest itself never feels crowded. Visitors quickly disperse. As a fitting reflection of our community, recreationists in McDonald Forest are generally peaceful and friendly, enjoying their good fortune at having such a great area to get out in.

Note: There is an excellent recreation map of the McDonald Forest and north Corvallis area. It is produced by Sky Island Graphics and is available at local book and sporting good stores. To become intimately familiar with McDonald Forest and its myriad of roads and trails, I highly recommend it as a companion to this guide.

McDonald Forest:
Oak Creek Area

This is a popular entry point into the western-most part of McDonald Forest. All outings here start along the cool and shady Oak Creek riparian corridor. All seasons are nice here, but in spring the wildflowers are especially wonderful. As this is a theme 4 level of management by the College of Forestry, the forest is diverse and generally pleasing to travel through. Except for the Homestead Trail, all routes here climb substantially. Dimple Hill offers an excellent view of Corvallis and the Willamette Valley and McCulloch Peak has a yet higher view. The Oak Creek Biology Lab adjacent to the parking area is operated by the OSU Department of Fisheries and Wildlife. They and the College of Forestry regularly conduct research projects in the area on topics such as monitoring stream flow in the Oak Creek watershed and studying the riparian zone.

To get there: The following trails are all reached from the Oak Creek access. Follow Oak Creek Dr. west from the Harrison Blvd./53rd St./Walnut Blvd./Oak Creek Dr. junction for 2 miles to the junction with Cardwell Hill Dr. Veer right and follow Oak Creek Dr. 1 more mile to the gate at the Oak Creek Biology Lab. Adequate parking is at the gate or along the end of the road.

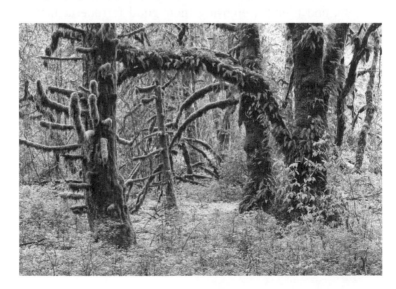

Trail 8. Homestead Trail

Length: 1.6-mile loop • **Elevation gain:** 120 feet
Difficulty: Easy • **Trail uses:** Foot, bike, horse
Trail surface: Gravel, trail muddy in spots during rainy
  weather
Seasonal closures: Open year round
Managing agency: OSU College of Forestry

The Homestead Trail Loop in the Oak Creek drainage is the only trail in the west side of McDonald Forest that does not do some significant climbing and, thus, it makes an excellent loop for walking dogs or introducing young children to the natural world. Spring arrives beautifully in this riparian area with an abundance of trillium, bleeding hearts, violets, and camas. Following that display, in May deep blue/purple delphinium make an absolutely fantastic showing along Oak Creek, reaching over 4 feet tall and then joined by equally tall cow parsnip. The Homestead Trail starts and finishes at the gate at the end of Oak Creek Rd.

As with most loops, it can be done in either direction. I suggest counter-clockwise, starting on the road and finishing with the nicest stretch, which is the Homestead Trail itself. Proceed straight north from the gate on Rd. 600, the Patterson Rd. In 0.5 mile take the first left on Rd. 6020, then immediately left again on Rd. 6021. All left turns will put you on the Homestead Trail for a delightful and gradually downhill finish over Oak Creek and back to the parking area.

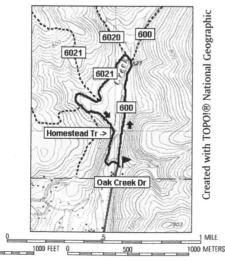

Created with TOPO!® National Geographic

Trail 9. Extendo and Uproute Trails

Length: 4.3-mile loop • Elevation gain: 690 feet
Difficulty: Moderate • Trail uses: Foot, bike, horse
Trail surface: Gravel, packed earth. Extendo Trail
   muddy during rainy weather
Seasonal closures: Uproute Trail—open year round,
   Extendo Trail—closed to bikes and horses 11/1 to 4/15
Management agency: OSU College of Forestry

This loop utilizes forest roads and trails and can be done in a few different ways, depending on preference and trail conditions. The loop passes through generally attractive forest with views limited to adjacent tree-covered ridges, which can be especially interesting in fall and winter when clouds and fog may cloak the steep hillsides. It is mostly shaded during the warm months. The loop starts and finishes from the gate at the end of Oak Creek Rd.

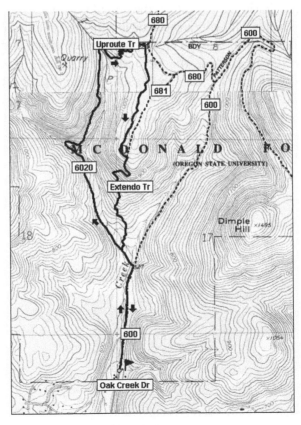

Created with TOPO!® National Geographic

The route I describe is a clockwise loop with two additional options for coming back down. Proceed straight north from the gate on Rd. 600. In 0.5 mile, turn left on Rd. 6020. Pass the bottom of Extendo Trail and continue on Rd. 6020 as it winds up, getting narrower and rougher, for close to 2 miles to its end. The Uproute Trail picks up here to prevent this from being a dead end. The well-graveled trail climbs steadily for 0.3 miles, topping out on Rd. 680. From this junction, loop back down on the Extendo Trail for 1.5 miles. This trail is steep in places and is favored by mountain bikers for its technical difficulty. Unfortunately, the steepness of this old horse route and the heavy clay soil, combined with the downhill zeal of mountain bikers, have created a lot of trail damage. The College of Forestry is, however, working to improve conditions on this trail while still allowing bikers to work on their technical skills. From the bottom of Extendo, turn left on Rd. 6020 and then right on Rd. 600 back to the gate.

Another option for the return journey is to start down Rd. 680 and in 0.25 mile turn right on Rd. 681. In about 0.5 mile, this old road will connect with the lower half of Extendo Trail; follow the trail 0.77 miles downhill to Rd. 6020. Turn left and then right on Rd. 600 back to the gate. The final option is to take all roads back down, which in the wet months is a good choice. Take Rd. 680 for about 0.5 mile to its junction with the main Oak Creek Rd. 600 and descend another 1.5 miles back to the Oak Creek gate.

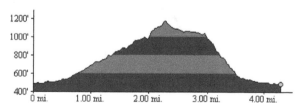

Created with TOPO!® National Geographic

Trail 10. Oak Creek to Dimple Hill

Length: 7 miles round trip • **Elevation gain:** 1,000 feet
Difficulty: Moderate to difficult • **Trail uses:** Foot, bike, horse
Trail surface: Gravel
Seasonal closures: Open year round
Management agency: OSU College of Forestry

This route to Dimple Hill is almost all on graveled road through attractive deciduous and Douglas-fir forest, gaining just over 1,000 feet and topping out on the open knoll with tremendous views. Some local runners and hikers make this round-trip jaunt weekly, and mountain bikers ride up it regularly as part of a longer forest ride. It is a good steady up-hill climb for those who like a good steady up-hill climb. The road is open and in good shape all year and any day is a fine day for a trip up Dimple Hill. The forest in this area is always lovely and the view from the top always satisfying.

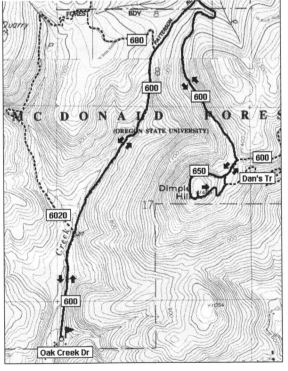

Oak Creek Area • Oak Creek to Dimple Hill

Created with TOPO!® National Geographic

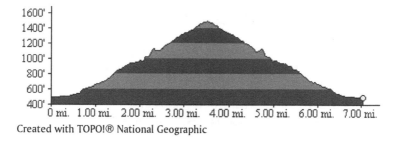
Created with TOPO!® National Geographic

Proceed straight north from the gate on Rd. 600, the Patterson Rd., past the Rd. 6020 and the Rd. 680 junctions. The road makes a sharp switchback and continues climbing to a saddle and four-way junction at mile 3. Turn right here on Rd. 650 for another 0.5 mile to the top. As a slight variation for the return trip, start down Dan's Trail to the east from the large boulder. In about 0.10 mile, turn left on a short connector trail that will take you back to Rd. 650. Turn right and then left on Rd. 600 for the long descent back to the trailhead. Though most hikers and runners return to the Oak Creek trailhead, bikers or long-distance runners can continue down Dan's Trail and back to Corvallis, or continue east on Rd. 600 to the Lewisburg Saddle, and on to Peavy Arboretum.

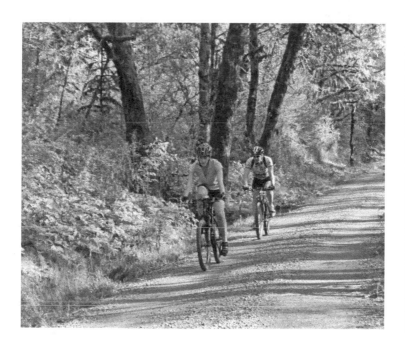

Trail 11. Oak Creek to McCulloch Peak

Length: 9.3-mile loop • **Elevation gain:** 1,900 feet
Difficulty: Difficult • **Trail uses:** Foot, bike, horse
Trail surface: Gravel
Seasonal closures: Open year round
Management agency: OSU College of Forestry

This loop proceeds mostly on forest roads from the Oak Creek trailhead at about the lowest point in the forest (480 feet) to the top of McCulloch Peak, which is the highest point in McDonald Forest at 2,155 feet. It is not a gentle route, and passes through some harvest areas, but makes for excellent uphill endurance training. The view from the top is outstanding and there is even a bench to sit and enjoy it from.

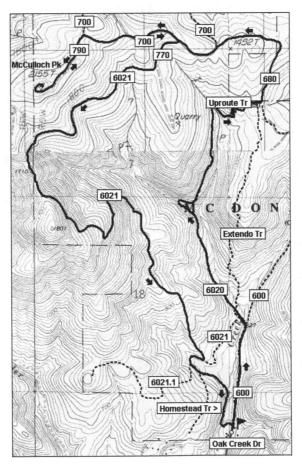

Created with TOPO!® National Geographic

Proceed straight north from the gate on Rd. 600, the Patterson Rd. In 0.5 mile turn left on Rd. 6020. Pass the bottom of Extendo Trail and continue on Rd. 6020 as it winds up, getting narrower and rougher, for close to 2 miles to its end. The Uproute Trail picks up here to prevent this from being a dead end. The well-graveled trail climbs steadily for 0.3 miles, topping out on Rd. 680. Turn left on Rd. 680 and continue climbing. At the junction with Rd. 700 from Soap Creek, keep left and keep on climbing. Stay on Rd. 700, noting the Rd. 770 junction for the route down. Turn left on Rd. 790. This last 0.5 mile to the top is the most pleasant as the uphill grade modifies and you pass through forest that has been left undisturbed for a while. The road ends at the top of McCulloch Peak. The impressive view to the south looks straight down on to the OSU sheep pastures and beyond.

The shortest way down is to retrace the route you came up; the loop described here makes for a somewhat longer, but more varied, trip back. Return to the junction with Rd. 770 and turn right onto it, and then right again on Rd. 6021. Except for one more climb, it is all down hill for close to 3 miles, passing through pleasing open forest. At the junction with Rd. 6021.1, you are on the Homestead Trail loop. Turn right, then left, then left again onto the Homestead Trail for a fine finish back to the Oak Creek parking area.

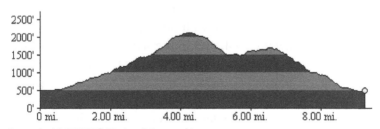

Created with TOPO!® National Geographic

McDonald Forest:
Jackson Creek Area

This is another popular area in the forest and many Corvallis residents can reach it readily and without driving to an access point. It is hilly terrain and many loops are possible between Dan's Trail, Horse Trail, forest roads in the area, and Chip Ross Park. The high point is Dimple Hill. This area is predominantly theme 4 level of management by the College of Forestry, so it is pleasant to recreate in.

The original Jackson homestead was located in the Jackson Valley where Dan's Trail, Horse Trail, and Rd. 612 converge. The house that is there today is a private residence owned by the College of Forestry. Jackson and Frazier creeks flow out of McDonald Forest, across Crescent Valley, and into the Jackson Frazier Wetlands, one of the last intact wetlands in the Willamette Valley. It is crucial to the survival of this wetland that these two creeks flow freely and that the impacts of logging, farming, and increasing urbanization be monitored and minimized.

Dan's Trail is, without a doubt, one of the nicest trails in the Corvallis area. It is close to town, well constructed and maintained, and reaches an excellent viewpoint on the top of Dimple Hill. The trail is not too muddy in the winter and come spring, wildflowers burst forth from brilliant green. Summer is shady and generally cool, and in the fall the foliage is lovely. Much of the trail was built by volunteer labor in the early to mid 1990s. The trail is named after Dan Petrequin, a long-time McDonald Forest equestrian and avid trail builder who died in 1992. The trail can be conveniently divided into three unequal sections. The entire trail can be traveled round trip, or can be combined with sections of Horse Trail and forest roads to produce outings of various lengths. The official start of Dan's Trail is at an information kiosk at the west end of the Chip Ross Park trail system.

Horse Trail is the route out of Jackson Creek that equestrians have been using for decades. Parts of it were rebuilt in the early 1990s to make it a little more accommodating of a grade for those on foot or bikes. Like Dan's Trail, Horse Trail can also

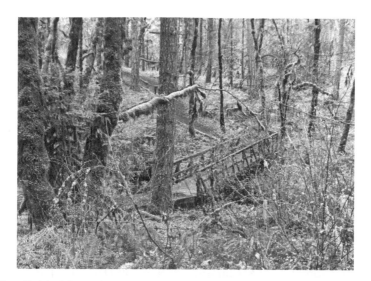

be divided into three unequal sections that can combine with Dan's Trail and forest roads to make a number of routes. The loops described here make Horse Trail the downhill portion.

To get there: There are two accesses to this part of McDonald Forest with available parking. The primary one is from Chip Ross Park, where the following trail descriptions start and finish from. From Walnut Blvd. take Highland Dr. north for 0.9 miles. Turn left on Lester Ave. The trailhead is in 0.7 miles, at the end of the road.

Secondary access is also being developed at the time of this printing from the top of 29th St. From Walnut Blvd., head north for 1 mile to the information kiosk and roadside parking for Timberhill Open Space. From the kiosk, take the left trail fork, heading north and then west. Pass through the upper portion of the Timberhill development, which is undergoing habitat restoration. Pass an old unofficial trail to the water tower and then come to a signed McDonald Forest connector trail on the right. Take this trail up to Rd. 612. Turn right on Rd. 612 and then left, just before the water tower, to reach the official start of Dan's Trail. Alternatively, turn left on Rd. 612 to drop into the Jackson Valley to intersect Dan's Trail or get on Horse Trail from the bottom.

There is a third access to this area by foot, bike, or horse, but no vehicle parking, at the end of Jackson Creek Rd., which becomes Forest Rd, 612.

Trail 12. Dan's Trail

Length: 7.6 miles round trip • **Elevation gain:** 1,400 feet
Difficulty: Moderate • **Trail uses:** Foot, bike, horse
Trail surface: Gravel
Seasonal closures: Open year round, except from Chip Ross Park to Rd. 612 closed to bikes and horses 11/1 to 4/15
Managing agency: OSU College of Forestry

From the Chip Ross Park kiosk, head west on the lower trail for 0.5 miles to a junction with the official start of Dan's Trail. Follow the signs for Dan's Trail as it winds down through nicely thinned forest into the Jackson Creek drainage, passing a junction at 1 mile. Continue straight on Dan's Trail another 0.25 mile to Rd. 612. Cross Rd. 612 and follow the second section of Dan's Trail through an old orchard and mixed forest for another 0.6 miles. Cross on a bridge over a small pool of Jackson Creek and come to Rd. 612.4. The trail continues up to the left. This last and longest section of Dan's Trail makes long, steady switchbacks through attractive woods for almost 2 miles, finally arriving at the top of Dimple Hill for a well-deserved pause to look around. From here, retrace the route back.

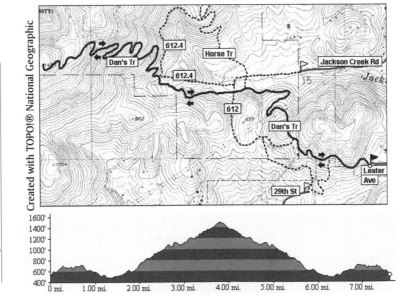

Trail 13. Lower Dan's Trail/ Horse Trail Loop

Length: 4.8-mile loop • **Elevation gain**: 845 feet
Difficulty: Moderate • **Trail uses**: Foot, bike, horse
Trail surface: Gravel
Seasonal closures: Open year round, except from Chip
  Ross Park to Rd. 612 closed to bikes and horses 11/1
  to 4/15
Managing agency: OSU College of Forestry

From the Chip Ross Park kiosk, head west on the lower trail for 0.5 miles to a junction with the official start of Dan's Trail. Follow the signs for Dan's Trail as it winds down through nicely thinned forest into the Jackson Creek drainage, passing a junction at 1 mile. Continue straight on Dan's Trail another 0.25 mile to Rd. 612. Cross Rd. 612 and follow Dan's Trail through an old orchard and mixed forest for another 0.6 miles. Cross on a bridge over a small pool of Jackson Creek and come

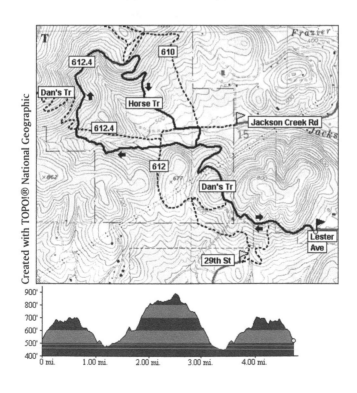

to Rd. 612.4. Continue straight ahead and uphill, following this rough road north for a mile to intersect with Horse Trail. Turn right on Horse Trail and descend into Jackson Creek valley for 0.75 miles, initially through thick forest and then through open meadow. Turn left on Rd. 612 and then right onto a spur trail crossing over Jackson Creek and connecting back into Dan's Trail. Turn left on Dan's Trail and retrace your earlier steps back to Chip Ross Park.

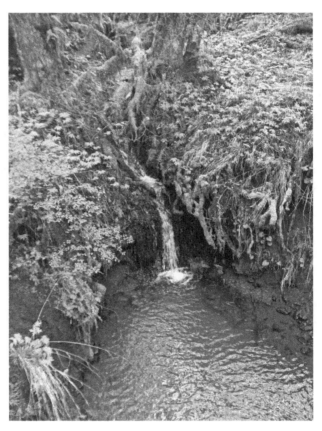

Trail 14. Upper Dan's Trail/ Horse Trail Loop

Length: 8-mile loop • **Elevation gain:** 1,450 feet
Difficulty: Difficult • **Trail uses:** Foot, bike, horse
Trail surface: Gravel
Seasonal closures: Open year round, except from Chip
   Ross Park to Rd. 612 closed to bikes and horses 11/1
   to 4/15
Managing agency: OSU College of Forestry

From the Chip Ross Park kiosk, head west on the lower
trail for 0.5 miles to a junction with the official start of Dan's
Trail. Follow the signs for Dan's Trail as it winds down through
nicely thinned forest into the Jackson Creek drainage, passing a
junction at 1 mile. Continue straight on Dan's Trail another 0.25
mile to Rd. 612. Cross Rd. 612 and follow Dan's Trail through
an old orchard and mixed forest for another 0.6 miles. Cross
on a bridge over a small pool of Jackson Creek and come to Rd.
612.4. The trail continues up to the left. This last and longest

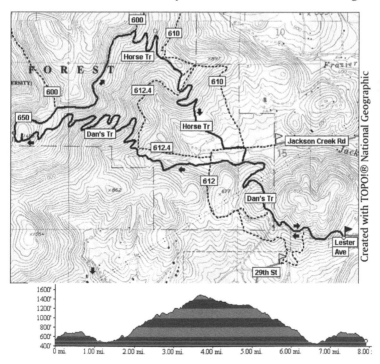

section of Dan's Trail makes long, steady switchbacks through attractive woods for almost 2 miles, finally arriving at the top of Dimple Hill for a well-deserved pause to look around.

From the top start down Rd. 650. At the four-way junction turn right on Rd. 600 and gently descend for close to 1 mile. Turn right down into the upper section of Horse Trail and switchback down, staying right, and on the trail, past a couple lefts out to Rd. 610. Horse Trail then crosses Rd. 612.4 and continues down into the Jackson Creek valley. Turn left on Rd. 612 and then right onto a spur trail crossing over Jackson Creek and connecting back into Dan's Trail. Turn left on Dan's Trail and retrace your earlier steps back to Chip Ross Park.

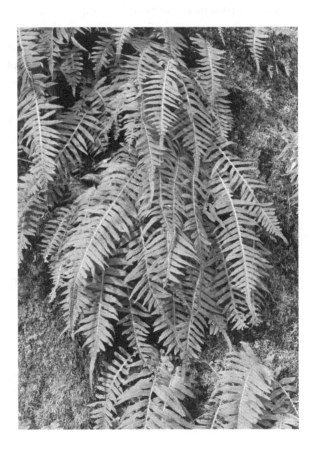

McDonald Forest:
Lewisburg Saddle Area

The Lewisburg Saddle is a low spot along the ridge separating Crescent Valley and Soap Creek Valley. This is a very popular access into the forest, particularly on weekends, but there are immediately four directions to head out in so there is plenty of space for all. Traveling west towards Dimple Hill takes one through diverse, theme 4 forest that is generally attractive and pleasant. Traveling east along Vineyard Mountain is through theme 2 forest which is periodically harvested and can feel less welcoming, but is favored for its near 7-mile loop with a moderate grade. The short Old Growth Trail through a small parcel of forest reserve is a treat.

To get there: These trail and forest road outings can all be reached from the trailhead at the crest of Sulphur Springs Rd. From Walnut Blvd., follow Highland Dr. north for 2.5 miles to the stop sign at Lewisburg Rd. Turn left and in 0.5 mile veer right on Sulphur Springs Rd. for another 1.5 miles to the top. Parking is on both sides of the road.

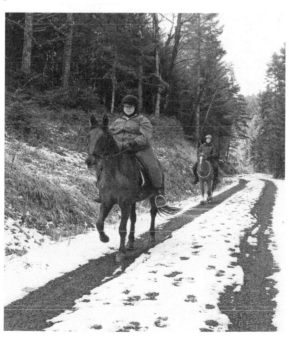

Trail 15.
Lewisburg Saddle to Dimple Hill

Length: 4.8 miles round trip • Elevation gain: 545 feet
Difficulty: Moderate • Trail uses: Foot, bike, horse
Trail surface: Gravel
Seasonal closures: Open year round
Managing agency: OSU College of Forestry

This is the gentlest way to the top of Dimple Hill. It is 1 mile shorter each way than coming up from Oak Creek and gains only a little more than half the elevation. It is a continuation of the Patterson Rd. from Oak Creek and is in good shape year-round. The route is mostly shaded in the summer, lovely in the fall, and always brisk in the winter. There are views of the adjacent hillsides and occasional glimpses south across Corvallis.

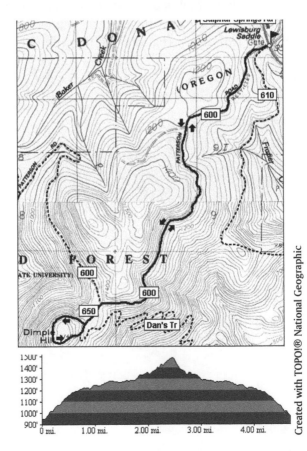

Lewisburg Saddle Area • Lewisburg Saddle to Dimple Hill

Created with TOPO!® National Geographic

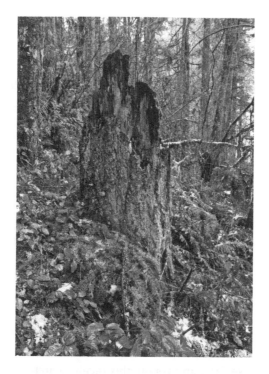

Head west from the gate on the west side of Sulphur Springs Rd. Immediately there is a junction with Rd. 610. Stay to the right on Rd. 600, the Patterson Road. The steepest section is the first 0.5 mile. The grade then moderates and contours nicely to a four-way junction at 2 miles.(Straight ahead takes you down into Oak Creek.) Turn left here on Rd. 650 and curve around to the top of Dimple Hill. As a slight variation for the return trip, start down Dan's Trail to the east from the large boulder. In about 0.10 mile, turn left on a short connector trail that will take you back to Rd. 650. Turn right and then right again on Rd. 600 and retrace your steps back to Lewisburg Saddle.

Trail 16. Lewisburg Saddle/ Horse Trail Loop

Length: 3.2-mile loop • **Elevation gain:** 460 feet
Difficulty: Moderate • **Trail uses:** Foot, bike, horse
Trail surface: Gravel
Seasonal closures: Open year round
Managing agency: OSU College of Forestry

If getting to the top of Dimple Hill is not a necessary goal, then this is a fine loop that enables you to enjoy the upper section of Horse Trail. Traveling in the clockwise direction gives a downhill start, a good climb in the middle, and a 1.5-mile downhill finish.

Head west from the gate on the west side of Sulphur Springs Rd. Immediately there is a junction. Take Rd. 610 to the left. Travel downhill through thinned forest. In 0.5 mile come to another junction. (Left takes you up for half a mile to a dead-end with a moderate view.) Keep right as you continue down through young forest. The road then climbs and where it levels out turn right into Horse Trail and follow this nicely switchbacking trail up for 0.64 mile. Turn right again when you top out on Rd. 600 (Patterson Rd.) and follow Rd. 600 down to Lewisburg Saddle.

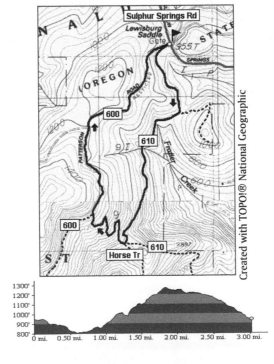

Trail 17. Vineyard Mountain Loop

Length: 6.5-mile loop • **Elevation gain:** 700 feet
Difficulty: Moderate • **Trail uses:** Foot, bike, horse
Trail surface: Gravel
Seasonal closures: Open year round
Managing agency: OSU College of Forestry

This forest road loop travels on two main roads of McDonald Forest in a long, narrow oval. It is a standard loop for many forest runners, hikers, and bikers and is a good choice during the wet months when many trails are muddy. In fact, I think it is most interesting when cloaked in winter clouds or fog. While it is hilly, the elevation gains and losses are not extreme, which contributes to the popularity of the loop. In years past it was truly beautiful; harvesting by OSU has increased in this area and portions of the loop now feel much more industrialized.

From the gate on the east side of the saddle the road immediately forks. The loop can be done in either direction and regulars all have their preference. The loop in a clockwise manner starts to the left on Rd. 580, Davies Road, with a downhill start, a downhill finish, and a long gradual climb in the middle. The loop in a counterclockwise manner starts to

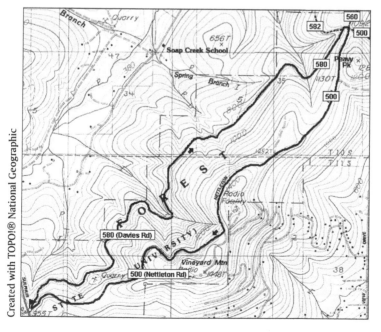

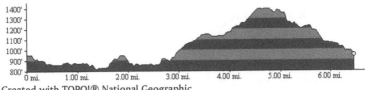

Created with TOPO!® National Geographic

the right on Rd. 500, Nettleton Road, with an uphill start, an uphill finish, and a long gradual downhill in the middle. The elevation profile is in the clockwise manner; start downhill to the left. The two roads meet at the halfway point where Rd. 500 continues on to Peavy Arboretum.

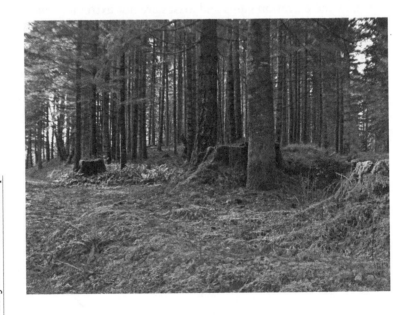

Trail 18. Old Growth Trail

Length: 1.6-mile loop • **Elevation gain:** 260 feet
Difficulty: Easy • **Trail uses:** Foot
Trail surface: Gravel, packed earth; trail is muddy in
  wet weather
Seasonal closures: Open year round
Managing agency: OSU College of Forestry

This short but beautiful trail passes through a relatively small preserved area of old growth in an otherwise heavily harvested section of McDonald Forest. This is notable low-elevation native forest, quite diverse in habitat with Douglas-firs that are over two hundred years old, towering maples, and a profusion of spring and early summer wildflowers. It can be done as a peaceful loop walk on its own or as a short and soothing diversion from the Vineyard Mountain Loop.

From the gate on the east side of the road, head left down Rd. 580/Davies Rd. The Old Growth Trail starts at a brown marker on the left, 0.4 mile down from the Saddle. The 0.5-mile trail drops down and then parallels the road, crossing a couple of bridges and climbing wooden stairs to rejoin the Davies Road. Turn right and follow the road back to the Saddle.

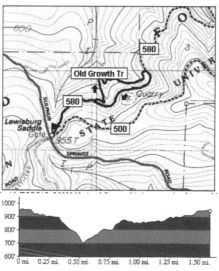

Created with TOPO!® National Geographic

McDonald Forest:
Soap Creek Area

The Soap Creek Valley lies north of Lewisburg Saddle. This northwestern corner of McDonald Forest is the least frequently visited by recreationists. It is managed by the College as theme 1 and 2 so periodic harvesting can be expected. Residents of this valley take advantage of the remote, well-maintained gravel roads to walk, bike, or ride their horses. Corvallis residents venture over the hill to recreate away from the "crowds" on the front side.

Years ago visitors traveled here to visit the healthful waters of Sulphur Springs. In the 1930s the Civilian Conservation Corps built a 20-acre recreation area with trails, campground, and picnic area, and it was quite popular. It became difficult to manage, suffered vandalism, and was dismantled in the 1950s. Little evidence of it remains, but there is an interpretive sign by the Baker Creek trailhead.

To get there: These outings are accessed on the north side of the Lewisburg Saddle off Sulphur Springs Rd. From the Saddle, continue over to the other side. In 0.7 mile there is an orange gate and limited parking for the 800 road system. For the following two trail descriptions continue 0.3 miles further, and turn left at the junction with Soap Creek Road. The Baker Creek trailhead and kiosk is in 0.2 mile on the left. The Soap Creek trailhead and kiosk is 0.7 mile further at an orange gate.

Trail 19. Baker Creek Trail

Length: 0.6 mile round trip • **Elevation gain:** 70 feet
Difficulty: Easy • **Trail uses:** Foot, bike, horse
Trail surface: Gravel, but the first part of the trail can
    be muddy in the rainy season
Seasonal closures: Open year round
Managing agency: OSU College of Forestry

This short outing follows along Baker Creek to an impressive beaver dam. In the mid 1970s an 80-foot beaver dam crossed the Baker Creek Valley just above its convergence with Soap Creek. It has been washed out and rebuilt more than once and today creates a very large pond, though the area is an ongoing work in progress.

From the trailhead, cross Soap Creek on the "new" bridge installed in 2004. When McDonald Forest lacked funding to rebuild the old bridge, they were able to recycle from a Benton County road this handsome 80-year-old bridge that could no longer handle large truck traffic. It easily accommodates forest visitors. Follow the shaded trail along Baker Creek for just 0.23 mile. At the junction with Rd. 800 turn right and come shortly to the Beaver pond. This is a quiet and peaceful spot and a fine place to observe pond life. Rd. 800 continues to the west, becoming overgrown, and eventually dead-ends. A few spur roads also become overgrown and dead-end on private forest land.

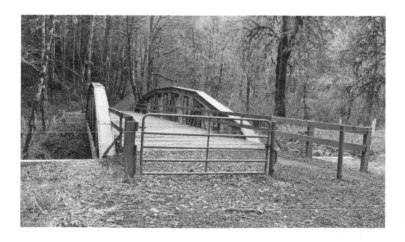

Note: Another option from this trailhead is to use the 800 road system to connect up to Lewisburg Saddle or the Jackson Creek area. From where the Baker Creek Trail joins Rd. 800, turn left on Rd. 800, then right on Rd. 810. Climb somewhat steeply. Where the road ends, the short but well-maintained Alpha Trail continues up to connect with Rd. 600. It makes possible a very long loop of the west side of McDonald Forest using the 600, 700, and 800 roads. Consult a McDonald Forest map for that loop as there are many unmarked and dead-end roads.

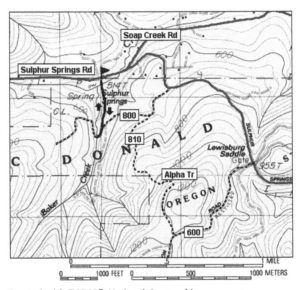

Created with TOPO!® National Geographic

Trail 20. Soap Creek to McCulloch Peak

Length: 7.7-mile loop or 9 miles round trip • Elevation
gain: 1,600 feet
Difficulty: Difficult • Trail uses: Foot, bike, horse
Trail surface: Gravel
Seasonal closures: Open year round
Managing agency: OSU College of Forestry

This route to McCulloch Peak through the more remote northwestern corner of McDonald Forest is a less-traveled alternative to climbing up from the Oak Creek side. It is all on forest roads and can be done as a demanding loop or an up and down on the gentler side of the loop. The trail description, map, and elevation profile are for a loop. Either way you can enjoy the nice woods in the Soap Creek drainage, have a commanding view from the top, and likely not see anyone else.

From the orange gate and kiosk, take the lefthand road (Rd. 700); you will start uphill right away, along the pretty and shady riparian zone of Soap Creek. In 0.8 mile, veer right on the faintly

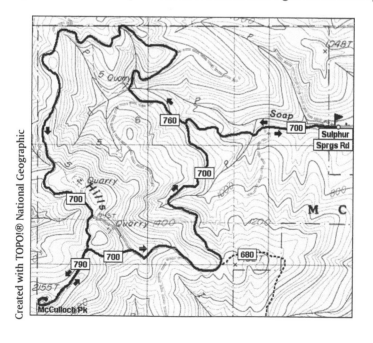

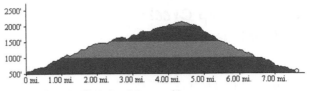

Created with TOPO!® National Geographic

marked Rd. 760. This road has some steep grades, but levels
out several times. Stay on Rd. 760 as you pass many dead-end
spur roads. At about mile 2.5, Rd. 760 becomes Rd. 700 and
follows a ridge south along the western-most McDonald Forest
boundary. At mile 4, turn right at the junction with Rd. 790 and
follow that to the top. To return, retrace your steps on Rd. 790.
To make the trip a loop, turn right on Rd 700 and follow that
steeply down. Stay on Rd. 700, veering left at the junction with
Rd. 680 coming out of Oak Creek. Continue dropping steeply,
passing the Rd. 760 junction that started the loop. Return to
the gate.

McDonald Forest: Peavy Arboretum

This is the most recreation-friendly area of the forest. It is managed by the College of Forestry at a level 4 theme and so is a mostly multi-aged forest with a variety of pleasing habitats. An extensive network of forest trails and roads makes for many great outings.

Peavy Arboretum area is the original 80 acres managed by the College. It was named for George Peavy, the first Dean. An arboretum was developed and now includes over 200 trees and shrubs native to the Pacific Northwest and elsewhere. A species index and map are available at the Badewitz Kiosk trail parking area.

Several buildings are located at the Arboretum. The field office for the College of Forestry is north of the Badewitz Kiosk and trail parking area. The Forestry Cabin is a quarter mile up Rd. 500 from the parking area. The original cabin was built in 1925 and then functioned as part of a Civilian Conservation Corps work camp. It burned to the ground in 1949 and was rebuilt in 1950. After the CCC disbanded, the Regional Office of the Oregon State Department of Forestry moved here.

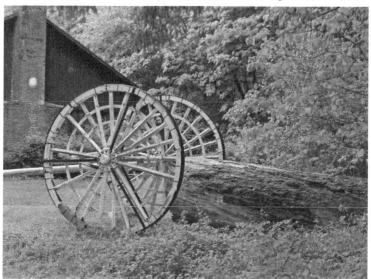

Old logging equipment beside the Forestry cabin

Peavy Lodge, at the Arboretum entrance, was part of their office complex. Built in 1948, the lodge has been extensively remodeled and is managed by the OSU Memorial Union for activities such as weddings, parties, and conferences. The Firefighter Memorial Shelter is dedicated to all who work to protect forest resources. The nine Willamette Valley ponderosa pines that surround the shelter commemorate the nine young Oregon firefighters who died in a wildfire in Glenwood Springs, Colorado, in 1994.

To get there: From Walnut Blvd. in Corvallis drive 3.5 miles north on Hwy 99. Turn left on Arboretum Rd. Continue north for 0.9 miles and turn left into the Arboretum. The road forks immediately and then again. Take the first left fork for all trails except for the Woodland Trail. Take the second right fork for the Intensive Management and Calloway Creek trails. Pass Peavy Lodge and park in the lot stright ahead. Keep left for the Forest Discovery, Section 36 Loop, and Powder House trails to the parking area by the Badewitz Kiosk where the road beyond is gated.

Alternatively, there is limited parking off Hwy 99, across from Adair Village at the gated Forest Rd. 540.

Trail 21. Woodland Trail

Length: 0.4-mile loop • Elevation gain: 10 feet
Difficulty: Easy • Trail uses: Foot
Trail surface: Gravel, packed earth
Seasonal closures: Open year round
Managing agency: OSU College of Forestry

This short and gentle nature trail was one of the first trails built in McDonald Forest. The interpretive signage on the trail highlights the interdependent systems of sunlight, water, air, soil, plants, and animals that make up a forest. A walk around this loop can remind us of these important relationships or introduce some of us to the basics of forest ecology. The trail passes through several habitats, including an impressive stand of incense cedars. Parking is behind Peavy Lodge and the loop starts and finishes on the east end of the lot.

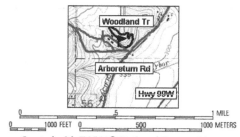

Created with TOPO!® National Geographic

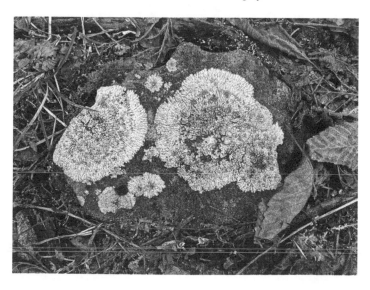

Trail 22. Forest Discovery Trail

Length: 1.7-mile loop • Elevation gain: 270 feet
Difficulty: Easy • Trail uses: Foot
Trail surface: Gravel, packed earth
Seasonal closures: Open year round
Managing agency: OSU College of Forestry

As the name suggests, this trail is one for "forest discovery." Interpretive brochures, usually available at the parking area kiosk, can guide and inform you as you walk along the trail and make for a more rewarding outing. Because this area once housed the State Nursery, there are some unusual trees and groupings of species that would not ordinarily grow here such as ponderosa pine and 50-year-old Port-Orford cedar. The loop offers a sample of several forest habitats. The trail starts about a hundred yards from the kiosk and parking area, back down the gravel road you came in on. A trail sign is on the right. The interpretive markers follow the brochure in a counterclockwise direction. There is a short but steep climb early on, and then the rest is gradually downhill. The forest trail emerges into the park-like setting of the lower Arboretum, not far from the starting point.

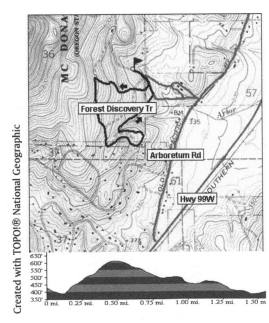

Created with TOPO!® National Geographic

Trail 23. Intensive Management Trail

Length: 1.5-mile loop • Elevation gain: 150 feet
Difficulty: Easy • Trail uses: Foot, bike
Trail surface: Gravel, packed earth
Seasonal closures: Closed to bikes 11/1 to 4/15
Managing agency: OSU College of Forestry

This trail passes through an area of forest genetics research. Primarily Douglas-fir is being studied here, exploring issues such as wood quality based on tree spacing, thinning, pruning, and planting different species together. There are also some ponderosa pine and brilliant orange-barked madrone along the way. As the name may imply, some of the forest is not especially attractive through here but the trail is gently rolling, very well maintained, and leads to the exceptionally nice Calloway Creek Trail. Parking is in the large lot just past Peavy Lodge to the right.

The trail starts at a sign at the end of the parking area. The first 0.4 mile passes through a variety of habitats in a short distance. The loop starts and finishes in a dark, plantation stand of very regular and tightly spaced Douglas-firs almost devoid of undergrowth. Take the right fork as the arrow points, and then take the next left at the Calloway Creek junction. Follow the arrows and signs for the Intensive Management Trail, crossing a few roads and again passing through changing habitats. At a three-way junction where Calloway Creek Trail joins back in, veer left. Complete the loop and return to the parking area on the 0.4 mile section of trail that you came in on.

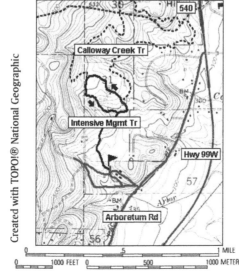

Trail 24. Intensive Management/ Calloway Creek Trail Loop

Length: 3.5-mile loop • **Elevation gain:** 250 feet
Difficulty: Moderate • **Trail uses:** Foot, bike
Trail surface: Gravel, packed earth
Seasonal closures: Closed to bikes 11/1 to 4/15
Managing agency: OSU College of Forestry
Other information: Favorite with runners

Calloway Creek is a truly wonderful trail that playfully curves and undulates through beautiful forest without gaining any serious elevation. The towering maples offer cool shade in the summer and superb fall color. Access is from the Intensive Management Trail. Parking is in the large lot just past Peavy Lodge to the right.

This loop starts at a sign at the end of the parking area. The first 0.4 mile passes through a variety of habitats in a short distance. Take the right fork at the first junction to make the loop in the counterclockwise direction. At the next junction, turn right onto Calloway Creek Trail and pass the backs of a few homes. Cross a forest road and wind through graceful forest, on

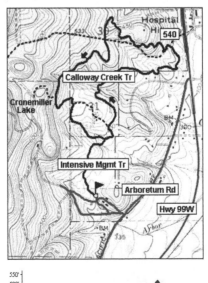

Peavy Arboretum • Intensive Management/Calloway Creek Trail Loop

Created with TOPO!® National Geographic

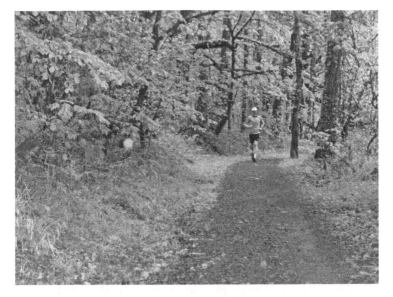

a well-constructed gravel trail that makes for heavenly running. Cross another forest road, Rd. 540, that is an alternative access point from Hwy. 99. This northernmost section of the trail climbs a bit and then continues in the same agreeable manner. It then crosses back over Rd 540 and ultimately crosses a bridge over Calloway Creek. Around the next corner is a junction. (Right takes you up to Cronemiller Lake where you can take the road down past the Forestry Club Cabin and back to the parking area or access the Section 36 Loop Trail (trail 25) and the steeper side of the Arboretum.) Turn left and then right on the Intensive Management Loop and then right again to return to the parking area on the 0.4-mile section of trail that you came in on.

Trail 25. Section 36 Loop Trail and Powder House Trail

Length: 4-mile loop
Elevation gain: 1,030 feet
Difficulty: Moderate
Trail uses: Foot
Trail surface: Gravel, packed earth
Seasonal closures: Open year round
Managing agency: OSU College of Forestry

These two trails combine to loop around the steeper western side of the Arboretum. The Section 36 Loop Trail is equally as pretty as Calloway Creek, and has a wonderful spring wildflower display. It is steeper, though, and climbs about 700 feet. The odd name comes from its location in Section 36, Township 10 South, and Range 5 West on the Willamette meridian. There is a marker on the lower portion of the trail designating this location. The extension to the Section 36 Loop Trail is the Powder House Trail which climbs another 150 feet to the high point in the arboretum and is worth the extra mileage. Its name comes from an old powder house built in the 1930s that stored up to 40 tons of dynamite used for logging and road building. The blasting caps to ignite the dynamite were stored a short distance away. The cap house and the foundation of the powder house are still visible along the route.

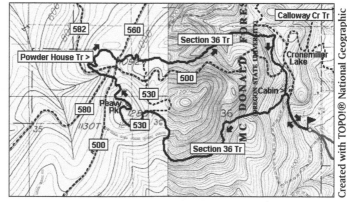

Created with TOPO!® National Geographic

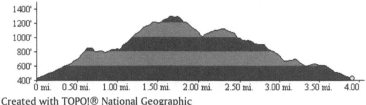

Created with TOPO!® National Geographic

This loop is only open to foot traffic; bikes and horses are not allowed at any time. Access is from the same parking area as Forest Discovery Trail.

Pass around the orange gate and head up the road for 0.25 mile to the Forestry Club Cabin. I describe it clockwise but, honestly, either direction works fine. At the cabin take the marked trail to the left. Cross the bridge and start up through pleasing mixed forest. A short descent on a series of steps breaks the uphill climb, but only temporarily. Notice some ponderosa pines as you pass. In 1928 seedlings from ten different locations were planted in this State Nursery to find a variety that would grow well here. Some did grow well and are still growing, while others died out. A little further up, notice a couple of huge trees, different from the rest. The lower branches indicate these Douglas-fir trees originated in a more open environment before thicker stands of the trees encroached; hence they are quite old. The trail gets steeper and darker before emerging onto forest Rd. 530.

If you are not including the Powder House Trail in your loop, then turn right here and travel down the road for 0.5 mile to the junction with forest Rd. 500. The Section 36 Loop Trail continues on the other side of Rd. 500.

If you are completing the entire loop, turn left and curve up the road to the hill top of Peavy Peak. Just ten years ago two memorial benches overlooked the valley to the east. While the benches are still there, the trees have grown and the view is hidden. The descent begins here. The trail winds down through pleasantly thinned forest. Follow trail signs as you cross a series of roads (Rds. 500, 580, and 582) in very short order. Just stay on the trail. The section of trail after the third road crossing travels through a drastic tree-harvesting site, but consequently affords quite a view to the north across the Soap Creek Valley and OSU's Dunn Forest. As the trail starts a brief

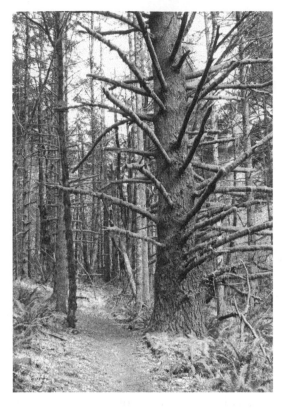

climb, there is a short fork to the right leading to the powder house foundation. The main trail continues left, entering the forest again, then dropping down and crossing Rd. 560. The old cap house sits here. The Powder House Trail continues down, crossing a bridge over a fern-filled gulley, to reconnect with Section 36 Loop Trail. Keep going down through beautiful old-growth forest. Cross a new and improved bridge rebuilt after the infamous January 2004 ice storm dropped a large tree that totally destroyed the old bridge. Continue down, more gently now, to Cronemiller Lake. Turn right along the lake and follow signs back to the Forestry Cabin and parking area.

Note: If another few miles through the lower part of the arboretum are desired, Calloway Creek Trail can be accessed from the other side of Cronemiller Lake.

Jackson-Frazier Wetland

Hidden behind suburbia in the northeast corner of Corvallis, lies a 144-acre natural area where many a visitor regularly comes to seek solace from the pace and noise of everyday life. Words can barely describe the magical moods that emanate from this obscure parcel of land. Whether one walks through this set-aside little world on a cold, foggy December day, during a fresh spring shower, at sunrise or sunset, the regulars can attest that frequent visits become habit-forming and one leaves feeling inspired and refreshed.

Jackson and Frazier creeks drain into this wetland from the northwest. A wetland is characterized by standing water or saturated soils in winter and spring, and is important ecologically as it purifies the water and soaks up rainwater to control flooding. A wetland changes throughout the year. In the winter there may be large ponds which recede to a slow-moving stream that may then dry to a cracked mudflat in the summer. Where once the Willamette Valley bottom was covered with wet prairie that the Native Americans burned regularly for food production, there is precious little of it left anymore.

Certain plants are adapted to live in a waterlogged environment such as this. More than three hundred species of flowering plants have been recorded in Jackson Frazier Wetland, including three listed as threatened or endangered (Bradshaw's lomatium, Nelson's sidalcea, and Kincaid's lupine.) More than seventy birds have been identified in this haven, including song birds, water birds, and raptors. We are fortunate to have this natural area to walk through, learn from, and enjoy without even having to get our feet wet.

In 1849 the land was first incorporated into a farm. It changed hands many times but was never intensely farmed due to the heavy, poorly drained soil. It was heavily grazed until the early 1960s. Its history of ownership and zone changes is long. Finally, though, in 1990, through foreclosure, Benton County assumed title and it was zoned as Open Space and Wetland.

Meanwhile, behind the scenes, local resident and OSU Emeritus Professor of Geography Bob Frenkel was envisioning what a wonderful resource for the community this land could be. A man of great dedication and focus, Frenkel is the prime mover behind Jackson-Frazier Wetland. From his first view of the property in 1978 through the "driving of the golden stake" to connect the 3,400-foot boardwalk loop in 1998, Frenkel led the way. Major funding for the materials was provided by the Environmental Protection Agency and labor was done mostly by youth and adult volunteers over four consecutive summers. Frenkel still leads the technical committee that advises the county on continuing to restore the wet prairie and protect its watershed. Fittingly, the boardwalk now bears his name.

When one sees the countless meadows paved over, hillsides deforested, lowlands built upon, and wetlands traded, it is refreshing and reassuring now and then to see one protected. Go forth and enjoy.

To get there: Jackson-Frazier Wetland can be reached from either Hwy. 99W or Hwy. 20, both of which have brown county signs directing one onto Conifer Blvd. Two blocks west of Cheldelin Middle School, turn north on Lancaster Street. Ample parking is at the end of Lancaster. A short concrete path leads eastward to the kiosk and the wetland entrance. A concrete path from the east also connects the adjacent neighborhood and Cheldelin School. The boardwalk is ADA accessible. Off-boardwalk access is only allowed by permit for educational groups and researchers.

Trail 26. The Bob Frenkel Boardwalk

Length: 0.8-mile loop • **Elevation gain**: insignificant
Difficulty: Easy • **Trail uses**: Foot
Trail surface: Wooden boardwalk
Seasonal closures: Open year round
Managing agency: Benton County
Other information: Bikes may not be ridden on the
boardwalk; lock them up by the kiosk. Dogs must
be on a leash. Jackson-Frazier can be beautiful in
the winter and especially on frosty-cold days, but be
aware that the wooden walkway can be very slippery
in the shade

A short distance in, the boardwalk splits and creates a
loop. Walk it in either direction; walk it in both directions. At
times you are in a thick tangle of shrubs and trees, only to
emerge in wide open wet prairie or shallow ponds. Each type of
wetland you pass through is home to unique plant and animal
communities. Try to tune out the hum of Hwy. 99 and other
sounds of civilization, and hear, instead, the songbirds, the
trickling of water, the rustling of grasses in the breeze. Don't
forget to look up, as you may spot a soaring hawk or other
raptor. Observe the islands of pussy willows jutting up nearby,
and in the distance. The protected wetland extends far to the
north and west of the actual boardwalk. Along the western side
of the loop, view the wetland's watershed of McDonald Forest

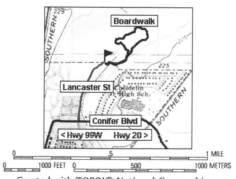

Created with TOPO!® National Geographic

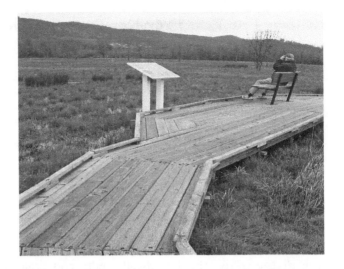

and Crescent Valley, as well as Owens Farm, another protected open space that someday may have a pedestrian connection from Jackson-Frazier. There are well-placed benches and several information panels along the way. Greater understanding fosters greater appreciation.

Bob's Boardwalk is a wonderful outing for small children as there is so much for them to discover. It is also perfect for wheelchair-bound folks.

Willamette Park/
Kendall Natural Area

Recent additions and improvements have done wonders for this friendly City of Corvallis Park and Natural Area, first established in the 1950s. Situated along the west bank of the Willamette River at the south end of town, this park now occupies 287 diverse acres. Willamette Park is a long rectangle with several paths of varying surfaces running parallel to each other. The sports fields and multi-modal path are in the middle, the river is on the east side and the restoration area is on the west side. With a variety of landscape features, trails, and facilities, this is a well-used park.

The south end has a large grassy area with shade trees, picnic tables, a covered picnic shelter, children's play equipment, and ball fields, all viewing the river. There is a small campground. A disc golf course is spread harmoniously through the woods and open areas. A paved multi-modal path connects residents of south Corvallis past the water-treatment plant, through the park, and on to downtown, OSU, and beyond. There are benches along the river where one can just sit and watch the Willamette make its way from its headwaters in the Cascades, north through the Willamette Valley to where it will join the Columbia River in Portland, and then on to the ocean. It is a good place to observe birds and other river life. The paved path is wheelchair accessible.

The north end of the park is Willamette Boat Landing, developed with a grant from the Oregon State Marine Board. Crystal Lake Sports Park is a large complex of soccer and baseball fields. The 80-acre Kendall Natural Area surrounding the sports fields and extending to the south is a riparian and mixed-woodland site of native plant restoration.

To get there: To reach Willamette Park's north entrance from Hwy. 99W (3rd St.), travel east on Crystal Lake Dr. for 0.5 mile, turn left on Fischer Lane. The road ends at a large parking area. To reach the south entrance, travel south on Hwy. 99W (3rd St.) 1.1 miles from Avery Ave./Crystal Lake Dr. and turn left at Goodnight Ave. The park is at the end of the road.

Trail 27. Willamette Park/ Kendall Natural Area Loop Trail

Length: 2.6-mile loop • **Elevation gain:** insignificant
Difficulty: Easy • **Trail uses:** Foot, bike
Trail surface: Paved, packed earth, bark
Seasonal closures: Open year round
Managing agency: City of Corvallis
Other information: A popular dog-walking area. Kiosks at both ends have a map describing the off-leash/on-leash areas and seasons. The non-paved trails allow dogs to exercise off-leash all year

The loop may start at either end and has many options depending on trail conditions, weather, and preference. This description begins at the southern end of the park and makes a counterclockwise loop around the perimeter. From the parking area closest to the river, proceed north on the paved path. At the first fork, branch off to the right on the dirt trail and travel through this shady riparian woodland corridor. In spring the many shades of green are exceptionally vibrant, while the wildflower display includes fringe cups, larkspur, cow parsnip, and many others. Late summer brings good blackberry picking along here and the path is full of leaves during fall. Attempting

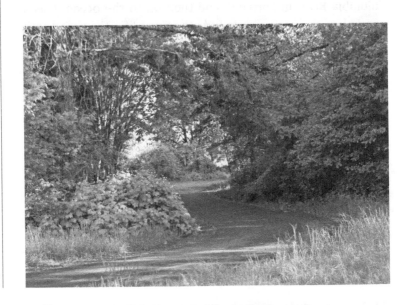

Willamette Park/Kendall Natural Area Loop Trail

to drown out city sounds is a chorus of songbirds, geese, and ducks along the river. Various side paths to the right lead to the broad river bank and one such path continues parallel to the main path, only closer along the river. Small side paths also lead off to the left and connect to a parallel bark-covered trail closer to the sports fields. This bark path is a good option when the main dirt trail is muddy. Close to the northern end of the park the trail forks. The right fork heads to the boat ramp and parking lot. Left takes you to the adjacent park kiosk. Either way works. From the kiosk, head west on the paved path away from the river, passing along the northern edge of the sports fields. Pick up a subtle dirt path and enter the restoration area. Proceed south through this open habitat. Curve east briefly along the southern edge of the sports fields and continue south paralleling the paved path. At a wall of blackberry veer right, then left, and re-enter the cool shady woodlands. Listen, perhaps, for the sociable clink of discs landing in the chained baskets. You are back at the south end of the park.

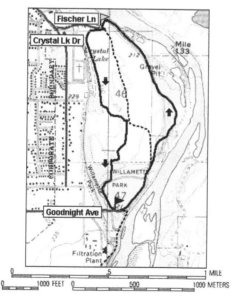

Created with TOPO!® National Geographic

Avery Park

This 75-acre wooded park in south-central Corvallis was my first introduction to the well-cared-for parks in this town .There is something for everyone here. Many residents use this park regularly and visitors to Corvallis can get a sample of the qualities that make Corvallis such a livable community.

The history of Avery Park dates to 1937 with the first of three land purchases that make up the park. It was named Avery Park for Joseph and Martha Avery, original owners of the land claim that the park is part of. The first bridge over the Marys River on 15th St. was built in 1941. The City of Corvallis and various community service organizations have been contributing to the park's development ever since.

Avery Park has a walking and running path that is described below. The wooded path and large expanse of grass make this a popular running area with OSU students, faculty, and the cross-country team, as well as middle and high school runners. Cross-country meets are hosted here, as are orienteering meets and local citizen runs and walking events.

The park has plenty of frolicking space and unique features for kids to play on including concrete "dinosaur bones," a historic 1922 steam locomotive, more traditional play equipment, and ball fields. The Avery House Nature Center at the east end offers environmental education programs for youth. There are several large picnic shelters for group gatherings, reunions, etc. that can be reserved through the City of Corvallis Parks and Recreation Department. The Corvallis Rose Society, in conjunction with Corvallis City Parks and Recreation, has developed an outstanding rose garden. The Corvallis City Parks and Recreation Administration offices are located at the west end of the park.

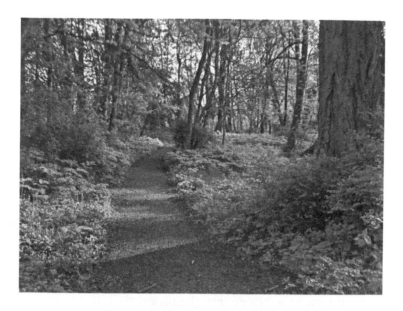

To get there: To reach the park from Philomath Blvd. (Hwy. 20/34), turn south on 15th St. and cross the bridge into the park. From Hwy. 99W (3rd St.), turn west on Avery Ave. There are several parking areas. The Corvallis-Philomath bike path crosses 15th St., so the park is readily accessible by bike.

Trail 28. Wildflower Trail/ Avery Park Loop

Length: 1.3-mile loop • **Elevation gain:** insignificant
Difficulty: Easy • **Trail uses:** Foot, bike
Trail surface: Gravel, packed earth
Seasonal closures: Open year round
Managing agency: City of Corvallis

The short but lovely wildflower trail at the west end of Avery Park can be combined with the rest of a loop around the park to make for a little over a mile. Runners do the loop repeatedly, or add on mileage from OSU, along the paved bike path to downtown, or west to Starker Arts Park. The loop may be accessed from anywhere in the park but the Wildflower Trail starts just over the bridge into the park from 15th St. Happily leave the pavement here, heading west along the banks of the Marys River through a shaded woodland. The trail is partly graveled and usable year round, though a bit soupy in places during the wet months. Come spring, it is a delightful wildflower garden. The first to bloom are the trillium lilies, followed by a blanket of yellow fawn lilies, violets, and deep purple larkspur. Next to show are saxifrage fringe cup, tiger lilies, the large-leaved cow parsnip, and wild-rose shrubs. These and others

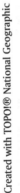

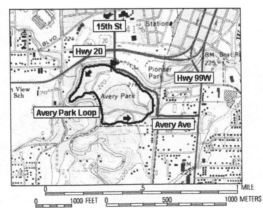

grow beautifully in the rich soil of this small peninsula which the Marys River loops around.

Just before the trail climbs a short rise, a spur trail leads to an old concrete and rock landing on the river where a concessionaire once rented canoes. This is a popular summer spot for folks seeking relief from soaring temperatures. The main trail passes the City Parks and Recreation Administration office and maintenance shops on the park road. Locals remember when the Marys River overflowed its banks during the flood of 1996 and a secondary river flowed through the park here. Historic winds have toppled many large, old trees throughout the park. Continuing on, enter the woods on a trail to the right. Several unofficial side trails lead to the river in various spots. All dead-end at steep, dense and eroded river banks and using them is discouraged.

The trail now follows along the southern boundary of the park, passing horseshoe pits and a community garden. Cross the park road leading to several picnic shelters. There is a compost demonstration site here, a joint project of City Parks, Corvallis Disposal, and the Avery House Nature Center. (Runners wanting a little more distance can add on 0.5 mile each way by running Allen St. south to the golf club.) If the grass is wet and you don't want to soak your shoes, follow the sidewalk along Avery Ave. Otherwise, cut across the grass by the picnic shelter. The Hull picnic table is an impressive single log slab that is 85 feet, 10 inches long. Pass the Avery House Nature Center, the steam locomotive, and go down the grass slope, past the dinosaur bones and ball fields. At this point, across Avery Ave., there is a covered interpretive display explaining the historic north-south Applegate trail and the settling of Corvallis (then called Marysville) by Joseph Avery in 1846. Finish the loop at the rose gardens, an extensive and well-tended collection punctuated by enormous cedars.

Marys Peak

We are all familiar with mountains that are jagged, snow-capped, majestic, and ... inaccessible to all but the most fit and skilled of mountaineers, while the rest of us must be content to view them from afar. Not so with Marys Peak. While it is a familiar landmark that makes for a nice western horizon from Corvallis, its distinct character cannot be realized by simply looking at it. And it need not be. It is less than an hour from Corvallis, and almost anyone can hike in this special place that has super trails and great views and is botanically unique and beautiful. A walk on Marys Peak is just plain good for the soul.

Marys Peak is the highest point in the Coast Range at 4,097 feet. On a clear day at Observation Point, views extend west to the Pacific Ocean, and east to the Cascades where the peaks of Mt. St. Helens, Hood, Jefferson, Washington, and the Three Sisters are lined up in their white cloaks. The Willamette Valley's cities, farmlands, and forests lay spread below. It is a wonderful place for residents to bring visitors, and if they enjoy hiking, that is even better.

Most of the terrain above 3000 feet—924 acres of the upper mountain—have been designated as a Scenic-Botanical Special Interest Area (SBSIA). The upper meadows host an outstanding collection of wildflowers. The East Ridge and North Ridge trails both pass through some of the best old-growth Douglas-fir forest in the Coast Range and then transition higher up into incredible stands of old noble fir. The Meadow Edge trail loops through both lovely meadows and beautiful noble fir forest. That these ecosystems are worth protecting becomes obvious as one also views the patchwork of industrial forest lands surrounding Marys Peak.

The weather is generally chilly on Marys Peak. It can easily be 10-20 degrees cooler than in Corvallis, windier and far wetter. If it is 40 degrees and raining in Corvallis, it is likely snowing on the mountain and this can be a great time to visit. When it is 90 or 100 degrees in Corvallis the shady forests on the mountain

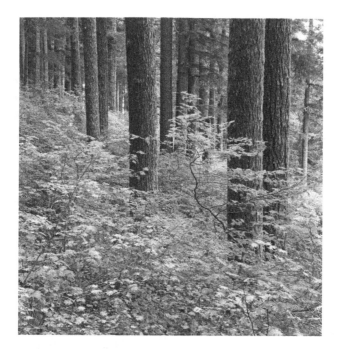

are blessedly cool. On a sunny day when the spring wildflowers are blooming there could hardly be a better place to be. On a crisp day in the fall the vine maple understory is lovely.

Marys Peak is no stranger to human activity. The Kalapuya Indians hunted, farmed, and conducted spirit quests on the mountain. The Forest Service once had a fire lookout near the summit and microwave and radio communication towers still exist, as unsightly as they are. The City of Corvallis Municipal Watershed comprises much of the eastern slope. Folks have been recreating on the mountain for decades. Amazingly, from the 1940s to the '80 s the Shriners would sponsor an annual trek where literally thousands of people would drive up to the summit for huge barbecues. That you are not the first to set foot on this mountain should not detract from your outdoor experience. It remains a wonderful place.

Most of Marys Peak is managed by the U.S. Forest Service and the Bureau of Land Management. A current Northwest Forest Pass, or equivalent, is required on all vehicles parked above milepost 5.0. An annual pass can be purchased at many locations or a day pass can be purchased at a fee station in the parking lots. Overnight camping is allowed only in the campground, which has six sites. Fires are only allowed in the metal grates

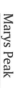

at the camp sites and in the picnic areas. Picnic areas are at Marys Wayside, Connor's Camp, Marys Peak Campground, and at Observation Point. Connor's Camp and Observation Point have wheelchair accessible restrooms. The road is usually open to the top from May 15th to October 15th, road conditions permitting; it is no longer plowed above the gate in the winter. When the gate is closed, parking is at Connor's Camp and access to the top is by foot, skis, or snowshoes on the main road or on the East Ridge Trail. Dogs must be kept on a leash.

To get there: To reach Marys Peak, drive 9.0 miles on Hwy. 34 from the Hwy. 20/34 split at the west end of Philomath to the Marys Peak Rd. at the summit crest between Philomath and Alsea. Turn right and begin the climb up Marys Peak. It is 5.7 miles to Connor's Camp (East Ridge trailhead) and the seasonal gate. The campground turnoff and trailhead for the Meadow Edge Trail are at mile 8.6. Observation Point and the Summit Trail are at mile 9.7.

To access the North Ridge trailhead, drive 1.7 miles west on Hwy. 20 from the Hwy. 20/34 split at the west end of Philomath and turn left on Woods Creek Rd. The paved road becomes gravel after 2 miles; the trailhead is 7.6 miles from Hwy. 20, at an orange gate.

Note: There is an excellent recreation map of Marys Peak. It is produced by Sky Island Graphics and is available at local sporting goods stores. It makes a good companion to this guide.

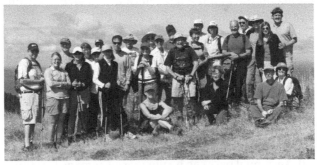

Hiking group at the summit of Marys Peak

Trail 29. Summit Loop

Length: 1.4-mile loop • **Elevation gain:** 385 feet
Difficulty: Easy • **Trail uses:** Foot
Trail surface: Forest floor, gravel
Seasonal closures: Open year round
Management agency: Siuslaw National Forest and
   Bureau of Land Management

The Summit Loop is the shortest trail on Marys Peak, but packs in outstanding views. Upon arriving at the parking lot at Observation Point, it is tempting to head right up the gravel service road to the radio towers on the top. I advise against this. The Summit Loop described here is far more satisfying and makes a nice figure-8, returning on the gravel road.

Soak in the view from Observation Point. The trail starts behind the kiosk, and heads south into the woods on the last stretch of the East Ridge Trail. Very quickly the trail will fork; veer right up the few steps and traverse gradually up through lovely mixed Douglas- and noble-fir forest as you wrap around to the south. Quite suddenly, you will leave the woods and continue contouring up through steep, view-filled wildflower meadows. At 0.32 mile cross the gravel service road and head into forest on the Summit/ Meadow Edge Trail. Immediately veer left at a junction to the summit. In a short 0.23 mile you will be there. If you find the radio towers unsettling, turn your back to them and—wow—what a panorama. Complete the loop by returning to the parking lot on the gravel service road.

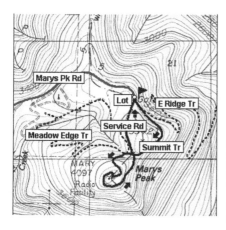

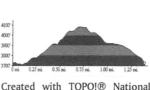

Created with TOPO!® National Geographic

Trail 30. Meadow Edge Loop

Length: 1.8-mile loop • Elevation gain: 460 feet
Difficulty: Easy • Trail uses: Foot
Trail surface: Forest floor
Seasonal closures: Open year round
Management agency: Siuslaw National Forest and
    Bureau of Land Management

This is a nice trail for families and visitors as it is not long and takes you through a beautiful and varied part of the Marys Peak summit area. In 1998, Eagle Scout Brian Collins developed a well-researched interpretive guide with corresponding markers for this trail. Brochures are usually stocked at the trailhead at the picnic area of the Marys Peak Campground. As with most loops, either direction works; the interpretive brochure and this description move clockwise.

From the picnic area by the campground follow the short spur trail in to the Meadow Edge Loop trail. Turn left and begin a gradual climb. A meadow gradually becomes visible on your left while lovely woods remain on your right. If nature had its way, the forest would slowly but continuously creep out into and, eventually, take over the meadows. During the hundreds of years before Euro-Americans came here, the Native Americans kept the meadows clear with regular fire for better hunting and food production. Along this transition zone you may notice

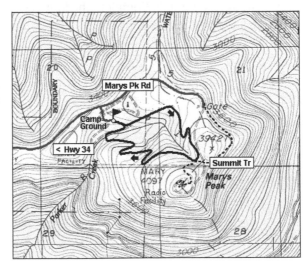

Created with TOPO!® National Geographic

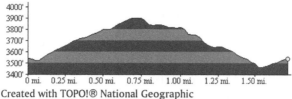

Created with TOPO!® National Geographic

how the Forest Service is attempting to preserve the meadows by removing the fringe trees.

Enter darker woods and pass the junction with the Summit Trail. The Meadow Edge Trail continues straight through dense, brown woods almost devoid of understory. After a brief but glorious stretch through a west-facing meadow, re-enter increasingly lush and verdant old-growth noble fir forest. In spring, the forest floor is a carpet of oxalis with many woodland wildflowers standing above: columbines, monkey flowers, iris, bleeding hearts, wood violets, and others. A wooden bridge crosses over the small and clear Parker Creek. The trail completes the loop at the spur back to the picnic area.

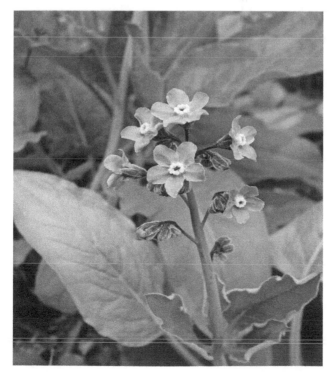

Trail 31. East Ridge/Tie Trail Loop

Length: 5.5-mile loop • **Elevation gain:** 1,200 feet
Difficulty: Moderate • **Trail uses:** Foot, bike
Trail surface: Forest floor
Seasonal closures: Closed to bikes 10/16 to 5/14
Management agency: Siuslaw National Forest and
Bureau of Land Management

A hike up the East Ridge Trail is a great way to arrive at the top of Marys Peak; you drive half-way up, walk the rest, and preserve the feeling of having reached the top on your own set of lungs. As a loop with the Tie Trail, it makes for a comfortable and very rewarding hike. The trail starts at the west end of Connor's Camp parking lot, to the left of the kiosk. The first step enters cool, green forest. Cross forest Rd. 2005. Climb gradually. The lower-elevation mixed forest with salal and Oregon grape transitions into a splendid cathedral of old-

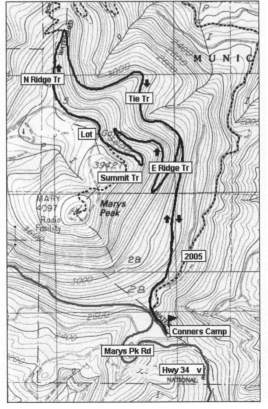

Created with TOPO!® National Geographic

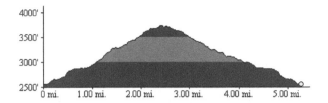

Created with TOPO!® National Geographic

growth Douglas-fir with vine maple, sword fern, vanilla leaf, trillium and others comprising the understory. Glimpses to the east over the Willamette Valley begin to emerge. At mile 1.04 is the junction with the Tie Trail. Switch back left and stay on the East Ridge Trail. The uniformly steep slope and soft forest floor leads up to rougher trail through rocky outcrops as it continues to switchback up the east side of Marys Peak. Walk under a large leaning snag (referred to as a widow maker), wedged between two stout firs, that has been there for at least ten years. Continue up through this splendid forest to the junction with the Summit Trail. If you are on a bike, you must proceed straight ahead to the summit parking area. If you are on foot, consider adding on the Summit Loop from this point. (Refer to Trail 29.)

To continue the loop with the Tie Trail, cross to the north corner of the parking lot and start down the North Ridge Trail (Trail 32). This is a gentle descent on soft forest tread for 0.66 mile to a bench and the junction with the Tie Trail. Turn right. Narrower and rockier than the relatively smooth treads of the North and East Ridge trails that it connects, the 1.2-mile Tie Trail is rustic and charming. Traverse gradually downward through a steep, primeval forest of old-growth Douglas-fir. Mossy seeps and springs cross the trail in several places. At the junction continue straight down the East Ridge Trail 1 more mile back to the start at Connor's Camp.

Trail 32. North Ridge Trail

Length: 8.4 miles round trip • **Elevation gain:** 2,165 feet
Difficulty: Difficult • **Trail uses:** Foot, bike
Trail surface: Forest floor
Seasonal closures: Closed to bikes 10/16 to 5/14
Management agency: Siuslaw National Forest and
Bureau of Land Management

The North Ridge Trail is the longest route to the top, and for those wanting a good, steady climb this is an outstanding hike. It is beautiful any time of year; however, this hike takes on a surreal quality in the clouds or fog. You may be fortunate enough to experience the utter silence, but for the haunting trilling of the varied thrush. The trail surface here is rougher than the East Ridge Trail and sturdy hiking boots are recommended.

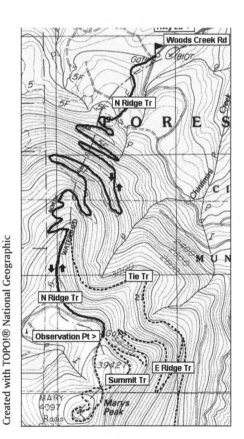

Created with TOPO!® National Geographic

The unmarked and undeveloped trailhead at the end of Woods Creek Rd. (which becomes Rd. 2005 at some unmarked point) has experienced dreadful resource damage done by vehicles going off-road. Walk around the gate across the road. In 100 yards a sign identifies the trail leaving to the right. The trail climbs from the get-go, but only for less than 0.25 mile before it levels and winds through idyllic forest thick with ferns, oxalis, trillium, and vine maple. Where an overgrown side path on the left leads to a lovely creek and connects to Rd. 2005, the main trail begins a series of switchbacks which make the steep slope quite accommodating to ascend. The trail climbs through large Douglas-fir, alternating between lush forest carpets of oxalis and vanilla leaf to areas devoid of undergrowth. In some areas severe winters have toppled the giant trees in a tangle over the trail, and it is no small task to clear the trail in the following spring. At mile 3.5 come to a bench and the junction with the Tie Trail. Continue straight ahead. The trail climbs more gently from here to the parking lot and Observation Point. Absorb the view and turn around here. The descent on the North Ridge Trail is perhaps even more beautiful than the trip up, as you are able to look down through the hemlock understory.

Or to continue on to the summit before returning, follow the sidewalk south to the start of the East Ridge and Summit Trail and make the Summit Loop. (Refer to Trail 29).

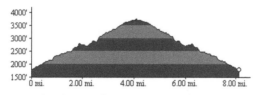

Created with TOPO!® National Geographic

Trail 33. North Ridge/Tie Trail Loop

Length: 8.8-mile loop • **Elevation gain:** 1,740 feet
Difficulty: Difficult • **Trail uses:** Foot, bike
Trail surface: Forest floor, gravel
Seasonal closures: Closed to bikes 10/16 to 5/14
Management agency: Siuslaw National Forest and
    Bureau of Land Management

This lovely forest loop starts and finishes at the trailhead on Woods Creek Rd. and bypasses the parking lot and popular Marys Peak summit area. It combines part of the North Ridge Trail, the Tie Trail, part of the East Ridge Trail and the gated forest Rd. 2005. It makes for a long year-round hike or a challenging bike loop between May 15 and Oct 15. If the day is glorious and clear, and the view from Observation Point too promising to pass up, forgoing the Tie Trail and, instead, taking the North Ridge Trail on up and coming down on the entire East Ridge Trail adds an additional 0.8 mile to the loop.

From the Woods Creek trailhead, walk around the gate across Rd. 2005. In 100 yards a sign identifies the trail leaving to the right. Climb for 3.5 miles to a bench and junction with the Tie Trail. It is mostly all downhill from here. Turn left and take the 1.2mile narrower and rockier Tie Trail to its junction with the East Ridge Trail. Continue straight and take the East Ridge Trail down almost to Connor's Camp. Turn left on Rd. 2005 and gradually descend for 3 miles, all the way back to the Woods Creek trailhead.

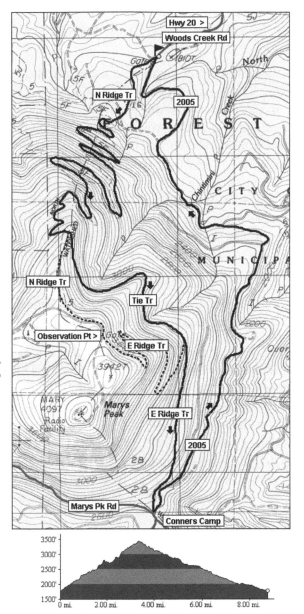

Coast Range Outings

The outings below are suggested as an introduction to the less recreationally visited Coast Range. Excluding Marys Peak, most Corvallis residents merely pass through the area between Philomath and the coastal towns of Newport and Waldport, enjoying the lush green corridor from their vehicles, but rarely exploring deeper. There is an abundance of public land between Hwys. 20 and 34. Much of it is part of Siuslaw National Forest, and some is State Forest. There are opportunities in this area for mountain bikers, in particular, to ride on quiet, graveled forest roads. These outings are west and northwest of Marys Peak and are accessed, not from the Alsea Hwy. 34, but from the straighter and more direct Newport Hwy. 20.

Note: Timber harvesting occurs in the Coast Range. The lush forest I describe in 2006 could be cut or thinned in the future.

To get there: The directions for the first two routes (Trails 34 and 35) start at the Burnt Woods Store. From the Hwy. 20/34 split at the west end of Philomath, drive 16 miles west on Hwy. 20 to mile marker 33. Do not be tempted 0.7 miles too soon and turn at the Burnt Woods Café. Turn left onto the Burnt Woods-Harlan Rd. 547.

To reach the start of Salmon Creek Rd. (Trail 36) travel 22 miles west on Hwy. 20 from the Hwy. 20/34 split at the west end of Philomath. Look for the green Salmon Creek Rd. sign on your left, and turn left here.

Trail 34 Sugarbowl Creek

Length: 5 miles round trip • **Elevation gain**: 670 feet
Difficulty: Moderate • **Trail uses**: Foot
Trail surface: Gravel, packed earth, wet
Seasonal closures: Open year round. Muddy during
   winter and spring
Management agency: Siuslaw National Forest

This outing is most suitable for foot traffic, as part of it is
wet much of the year. The trail travels down and back on an old
road, a portion of which is now an overgrown, albeit lush and
intimate, corridor of second-growth Douglas-firs, huge maples,
and a multitude of ferns.

Driving directions: From the Burnt Woods Store, drive south
on Rd. 547 for 0.5 miles and turn left on Shotpouch Rd. At mile
4, turn right at an unmarked road, cross the creek, and go up
0.4 mile to a four-way unmarked junction. There is not a formal
trailhead. Park here.

Continue down the middle road, opposite the one you came
in on. This historical portion of an old road to the coast is in

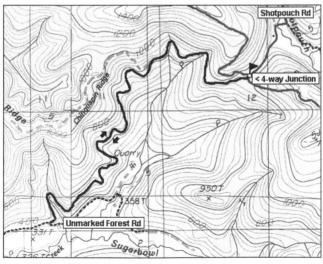

Created with TOPO!® National Geographic

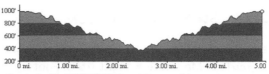

Created with TOPO!® National Geographic

good shape at first, but within a mile the road makes a turn to the left and rapidly becomes rutted and overgrown. It gets very overgrown, but manageable, for a short spell before reaching an unmarked forest road. Sugarbowl Creek is on the other side of the road. Turn around here and retrace your steps.

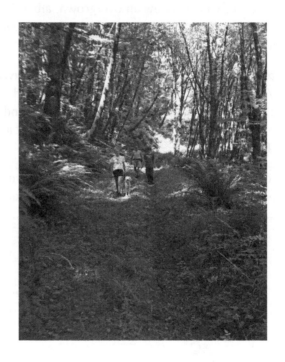

Trail 35. Strom Boulder Ridge Loop

Length: 7.6-mile loop • **Elevation gain:** 1,430 feet
Difficulty: Moderate to difficult • **Trail uses:** Foot, bike
Trail surface: Gravel
Seasonal closures: Open year round
Management agency: Oregon State Forests

This loop is on State Forest lands and is entirely on graveled forest roads. It alternately passes through thinned timber lands with far-reaching views of the forested carpet that comprises much of the Coast Range and more shaded miles through lush forest gushing with ferns and spring wildflowers.

Driving directions: From the Burnt Woods Store, drive south for 2 miles on Rd. 547. Turn right at the 2-mile marker on a gravel road. The loop starts at a junction 0.8 mile further. There is no formal trailhead. Park on the side of the road here at the start of the loop or 0.10 mile back there is another junction that could also be a suitable parking spot.

Make the loop clockwise by starting to the left on the signed Burnt Woods Ridge Rd. The gradual up-hill warm-up is short; the trail then becomes considerably steeper for 0.5 mile. It then moderates and rolls gradually down for a couple of miles along Strom Boulder Ridge. Stay on the main road until mile 2.3. At this unsigned fork, Wolf Cabin Rd. merges into Burnt Woods Ridge Rd. uphill from the left. Continue straight (right)

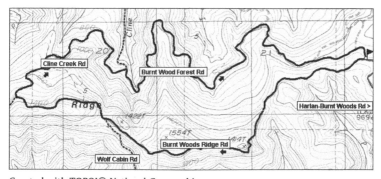

Created with TOPO!® National Geographic

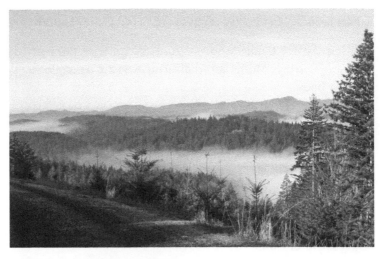

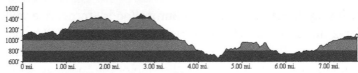

Created with TOPO!® National Geographic

for a short climb, then again roll along the ridge with nice Coast Range views as you pass around the headwaters of Cline Creek. Come to a signed junction on Burnt Woods Ridge Rd. and turn right on Cline Creek Rd. Continue mostly downhill for 1.5 miles to the final junction of this loop. Turn right on Burnt Woods Forest Rd. The final couple of miles gradually traverse and wind back up through sheltered woods to the start of the loop.

Trail 36. Salmon Creek Loop

Length: 12-mile loop • **Elevation gain:** 1,900 feet
Difficulty: Moderate to difficult • **Trail uses:** Foot,
  bike
Trail surface: Gravel
Seasonal closures: Open year round
Management agency: Oregon State Forests

This loop is also on State Forest lands and entirely on
graveled forest roads. It shares a common mile of Burnt Woods
Ridge Rd. with the preceding trail description. The trail travels
along two refreshing creeks, Salmon Creek and Wolf Creek,
climbs up onto Strom Boulder Ridge, and then loops back
down. You can decrease the length of the trail to 7.7 miles by
driving the Salmon Creek Rd. section; however, on a bike, this
would be a good section to ride.

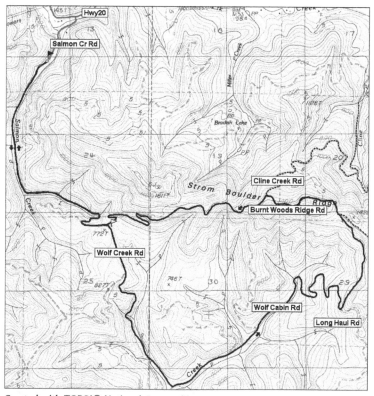

Created with TOPO!® National Geographic

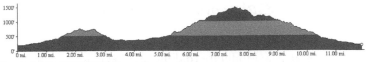

Created with TOPO!® National Geographic

Driving directions: There are no formal trailheads. To start the longer trail, from Hwy. 20 proceed about 0.5 mile on Salmon Creek Rd., past the private property. There is a large pull-out on your left to park. For the shorter trail, continue driving in Salmon Creek Road for 2.3 miles to the first junction and the start of the loop. Park here.

The first 2 miles on Salmon Creek Rd. follow the creek gently up through a leafy valley. A short climb brings you to the first junction. Turn right on the signed Wolf Creek Rd. Travel through thinned forest. At 4.2 miles, turn left on the unsigned Wolf Cabin Rd. (Wolf Creek Rd. continues to the right). Travel on the level along Wolf Creek. The road then climbs with several switchbacks. Stay on the main road and veer sharply left where Long Haul Rd. forks to the right. Continue up to the unsigned junction with Burnt Woods Ridge Rd. at mile 7.4. Turn left and travel up and down along the ridge. Keep left at the next signed junction on Burnt Woods Ridge Rd. (Cline Creek Rd. goes down to the right). Stay on this road downhill to the junction that started this loop. Veer right onto Salmon Creek Rd. and follow the creek back to your starting point.

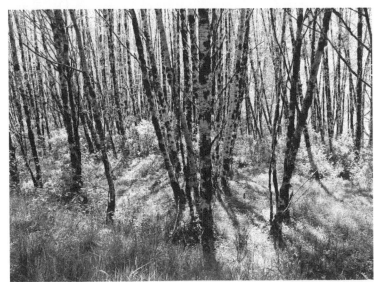

Beazell Memorial Forest

Beazell Memorial Forest in Kings Valley is widely regarded as the jewel of Benton County's park system. And rightly so; it is a beautiful spot. To know the love story behind the park is to more fully appreciate a visit there. Fred and Dolores Beazell worked together in Silicon Valley and married later in life. They had no children. In 1966, while still living in California, they bought this 586-acre property, which included an old farm, forests, fields, and open meadows. Fred and Dolores wanted to create a beautiful and peaceful natural environment where they could live quietly, observe birds and wildlife, help heal the land from past harsh logging, and nurture a young and growing forest. Though still living in California, Fred spent many a weekend coming up to Oregon to pursue his passion of planting trees on his property. They retired in 1981 and moved to Corvallis. They built a home on the property and Dolores enjoyed living there, especially feeding the birds. Fred was deeply devoted to Dolores, who passed away in 1993. As Fred continued to plant trees and care for his land, he began to envision the forest preserve that could evolve here. He began planning for the future of his property.

A long-time friend, Charles Ross, visionary of protected open space around Corvallis, nurtured the idea of leaving the parcel as a memorial to his wife. Fred became convinced that Benton County Natural Areas and Parks Department could best manage his property with the same conscientious stewardship that he had practiced for thirty-five years. He willed his property, appraised at $5.7 million, to Benton County. He did not want his land to be a financial burden to future taxpayers, and he reconciled to the reality of harvesting trees for the health of the forest, with the revenue covering the operating costs of the property. As his health was waning, he and Benton County Natural Areas and Parks Director, Jerry Davis, worked out the details for a self-sustaining public parcel, managed to promote a healthy and diverse forest, accessible to all, and to serve as a living memorial to his beloved wife, Dolores. Fred died in 2000. Some of his ashes are scattered among some saplings that were planted in his memory.

Benton County has worked hard to fulfill his vision, and Fred would be pleased. Beazell Memorial Forest is a well-respected model for environmentally sensitive forest management. It is certified under the Smart Wood Program, which assures that management meets stringent standards for environmental sensitivity, sustainability, and community and social concerns. Habitat restoration, in particular to preserve the oak woodlands and meadows, is an ongoing project. The park has a variety of habitats, including a lush riparian area along Plunkett Creek, Douglas-fir forests, oak savannas, and hilltop meadows with grand vistas. Benton County staff, along with community volunteers and other organizations, have constructed several miles of trails, with more to come. In addition, the 1930s-era barn on the site has been extensively remodeled into a forest education center. Beazell Memorial Forest opened in 2003, and is truly a gift to the community and a work in progress.

A visitor's first sight is the 1870s Plunkett house, one of the oldest dwellings in Kings Valley. Its exterior has been carefully restored to reflect its time period. You will find sufficient parking, restrooms, and picnic tables under the shade of a magnificent white oak.

All of the trail descriptions start at the forest education center.

To get there: To reach Beazell Memorial Forest head west from Philomath on Hwy. 20. In 4 miles, at Wren, turn right on Hwy. 223N to Kings Valley. Beazell is 5 miles north on the right.

Note: At the time of this writing, Bird Loop, South Loop, and Plunkett Creek Road are complete. The South Meadow/Plunkett Creek Loop and the Plunkett Creek Loop trails are expected to be completed by fall of 2006. Additional trails are anticipated.

Trail 37. Bird Loop Trail

Length: 1.2-mile loop • Elevation gain: 140 feet
Difficulty: Easy • Trail uses: Foot, bike, horse
Trail surface: Gravel
Seasonal closures: Open year round
Managing agency: Benton County

This short and gentle trail is ideal for bird watching or just a nice walk through a variety of habitats representative of the Beazell property. An excellent bird checklist has been produced in cooperation with the Audubon Society of Corvallis and is available at the trailhead kiosk.

Walk across and linger on the curved wooden bridge that spans not just Plunkett Creek but the whole riparian zone of the creek. Turn left for the Bird Loop Trail and parallel the creek for a short distance. Cross the lane to the Beazell house, currently occupied by a site host and not open to the public. The 1-mile loop begins in the meadow and can be enjoyed

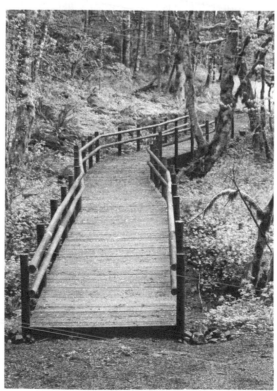

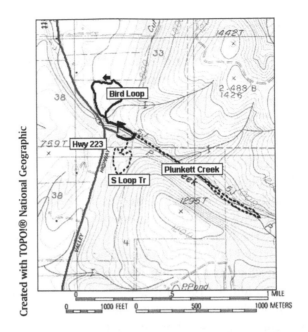

in either direction. This description starts to the right and proceeds counterclockwise. Very gently ascend through open grassland and second-growth Douglas-fir forest that are some of Fred Beazell's plantings. Remnants of old pasture fences are evident. Fred also planted some cedar trees in this area. At the north edge of the park, where the trail turns left, a bench offers a spot to sit and a view to the north across the adjacent property of open fields and stately oaks. Briefly pass through thick Douglas-fir. The trail now parallels the highway for a short distance and returns to the start of the loop. The two small footbridges were an Eagle Scout project. Return to the Plunkett Creek bridge. If you have more time, definitely consider a walk up Plunkett Creek (Trail 40) or at least the short South Loop Trail (38).

Trail 38. South Loop Trail

Length: 0.7-mile loop • Elevation gain: 150 feet
Difficulty: Easy • Trail uses: Foot, bike, horse
Trail surface: Gravel
Seasonal closures: Open year round
Managing agency: Benton County

This short loop is ideal for picnickers or others just wanting to stretch their legs. It is also the beginning of the South Meadow/Plunkett Creek Loop (39). The trail starts across from the education center at an information kiosk explaining how Benton County is managing the Beazell Forest for biodiversity, sustainability, and forest health. Cross the open area with remnant fruit trees from an earlier era and enter into cool, open woods that this trail will loop around. To the right is a side trail stepping up to an old dripping, moss-covered cistern that stored the ground-spring water for use by residents of the old Plunkett house. At the fork, turn left and make the loop clockwise. You may notice a lot of trees lying on the ground. After this area was thinned, many trees were toppled by the January 2004 ice storm. It was decided to let the trees lie and decompose naturally and build the trail around the debris.

The top of the loop is a grassy log-hauling road. If you are going on up the South Meadow Trail you will turn left here. Otherwise, turn right and, shortly, right again on the rest of the loop trail. Notice where large oaks have been "released" from overtopping Douglas-firs and where snags have been created for wildlife. Curve around the remainder of the loop, passing above the cistern. Left at the junction takes you back to the start.

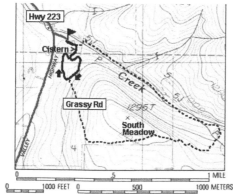

Created with TOPO!® National Geographic

Trail 39. South Meadow/ Plunkett Creek Loop

Length: 2.5-mile loop • **Elevation gain:** 600 feet
Difficulty: Moderate • **Trail uses:** Foot, bike, horse
Trail surface: Gravel, grassy road, packed earth
Seasonal closures: Closed to bikes and horses 10/31 to 4/15
Managing agency: Benton County

This loop climbs up a grassy log-hauling road past the south meadow to the edge of the Beazell property, drops down into the narrow Plunkett Creek drainage, and returns along one of the most beautiful riparian ravines in Benton County.

Start across from the education center on the South Loop Trail (38). Pass the cistern and take the left fork of the loop. At the grassy road, turn left and climb steadily for 1 mile past the south meadow to the high point on this side of the property. Turn right and wind down along the property boundary with views into the adjacent property which is managed quite differently. Descend through increasingly fern-covered mixed forest with towering maples. Cross a bridge over a tributary of Plunkett Creek and soon come to a junction. A right turn here will take you across Plunkett Creek and up out of the creek bed to the old Plunkett Creek road. Take the road here if you want to stay above the creek and view down into it. Otherwise turn

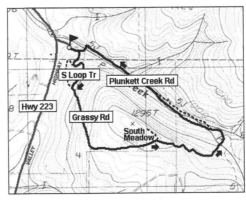

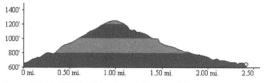

Created with TOPO!® National Geographic

left at this junction and take the more intimate trail down in the rich creek bed. This lower trail crosses two more bridges of Plunkett Creek and its side creeks, while meandering down the streambed, giving the visitor a wonderful connection to this extremely lush, lovely, and healthy environment. The trail merges into the old Plunkett Creek road and follows it 0.4 miles back to the start.

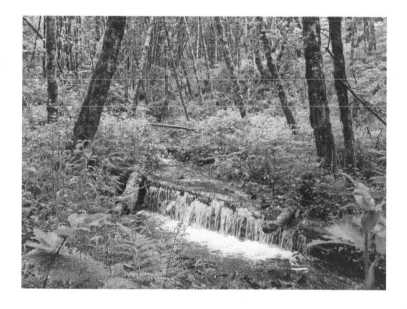

Trail 40. Plunkett Creek Loop

Length: 1.8-mile loop • **Elevation gain:** 260 feet
Difficulty: Easy • **Trail uses:** Foot, bike, horse
Trail surface: Gravel
Seasonal closures: Plunkett road open year round.
  Loop closed to bikes and horses 10/31 to 4/15
Managing agency: Benton County

This loop gradually ascends the now-preserved Plunkett Creek ravine on an old, but charming, log-hauling road, loops back part of the way on a delightful trail in the creek bed and then rejoins the road for a riparian loop that is a feast for the senses. It is extremely lush here in the spring with trillium lilies and bleeding hearts leading the show, followed by delphinium, cow parsnip, and so much more. Summer along here remains fresh and cool, fall highlights the vine maple and other hardwoods, while winter reveals the heavy mosses growing high in the leafless trees and the profusion of sword ferns in the understory. Plunkett Creek is a vibrant tributary of the Luckiamute River.

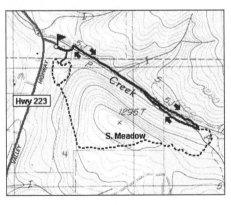

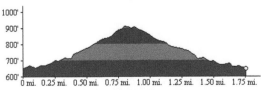

Created with TOPO!® National Geographic

From the education center, walk across the curved wooden bridge that spans the whole riparian zone of Plunkett Creek. Turn right and follow the old road. A forest shelter is planned for somewhere in this area. At 0.4 mile, pass the trail that you will come back on. At 0.8 miles, and just before a gate at the boundary with the neighboring property, turn right and switchback down into the creek bed. Cross Plunkett Creek and come to a junction. Left takes you up to the south meadow and on back to the education center. This loop turns right here and stays close to the creek to allow for a close-up passage down through this remarkable gulch. The trail merges back onto the road, where things look different going the other way.

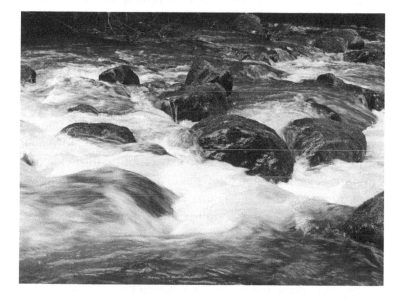

Fort Hoskins Historic Park

On a knoll overlooking the east-flowing Luckiamute River in Kings Valley sits one of Benton County's newest parks. A visit to this 130-acre park is an opportunity to appreciate the layers of history in this part of the county, enjoy a picnic, and take a nice walk as well. In a day outing to Kings Valley, one could also visit Beazell Memorial Forest, just down the road.

For thousands of years the Kalapuya Indians lived in the Willamette Valley. The familiar and sad story is retold here of early settlers skirmishing with the Natives and European diseases devastating whole tribes. Eventually the Indians were forced from their homelands onto two reservations, the Siletz and the Grand Ronde, where they were ill-equipped to survive and prosper. Fort Hoskins was established in 1856 to monitor traffic entering and leaving the newly established coastal Siletz Indian Reservation. The fort served as an important outpost for the Indians, for Oregon soldiers training for the Civil War, and for the settlers. The fort housed two to three hundred soldiers whose duties also included keeping the Secessionist movement in the central Willamette Valley from erupting into violence. The fort was abandoned after the Civil War in 1866, and the property was sold to the Frantz family that same year. They built a Gothic Revival-style house and replaced the barracks with farm structures and a blacksmith shop. The house is on the National Register of Historic Places and still stands on the east end of the park.Beginning in the 1970s many archeological studies were done and artifacts recovered that tell the story of years past. The property remained in the Frantz-Dunn family until Benton County bought it in 1992 with grant monies, county funds, and citizen donations. The park opened to the public in 2002. Today park visitors can enjoy a beautiful timber truss-style picnic shelter, a historic interpretive trail, and a 1.6-mile recreation trail.

The Indians used fire to manage their landscape. Regular fires encouraged the growth of important food plants, provided better forage for game animals, made for easier hunting and traveling, and lowered fuel loads to guard against catastrophic wild fire. Oak savanna and open prairie defined the landscape prior to European settlement. As steward of the park, one of Benton County's long-term goals is to recreate the habitat familiar to the Kalapuya, the soldiers, and the early pioneers. This is accomplished with periodic controlled burning, removing encroaching Douglas-firs, and reintroducing native plants.

To get there: To reach Fort Hoskins, head west from Philomath on Hwy. 20. In 4 miles turn right on State Hwy. 223N to Kings Valley. In 6.5 miles turn left on Hoskins Rd. Drive 2 miles west, veer right at a junction, and the park entrance will be on the right. The picnic shelter and restrooms are handicap accessible.

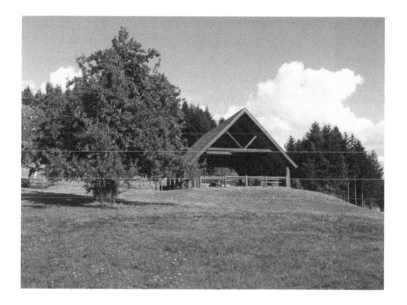

Trail 41. Fort Hoskins Recreation Trail

Length: 1.6-mile loop • Elevation gain: 315 feet
Difficulty: Easy to moderate • Trail uses: Foot, bike, horse
Trail surface: Gravel
Seasonal closures: Closed to bikes and horses 10/31 to 4/15
Management agency: Benton County

This short trail climbs the hill behind the picnic shelter and gives the visitor a look at the habitat restoration area, as well as fine views out over the Luckiamute River valley. The trail starts across from the restroom. Immediately you enter the cool shade of Douglas-fir woods. At the loop junction you may go either direction; this description turns left and makes the loop clockwise. Continue winding uphill through mostly Douglas-fir woods with bracken ferns and invading blackberries in the understory. As you get higher, the Douglas-firs give way to more open meadow and white oaks. From the short traverse across the top you can look down into the Luckiamute Valley

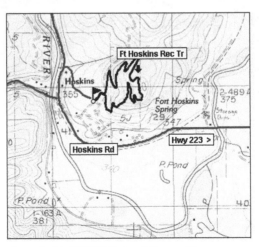

Created with TOPO!® National Geographic

and the industrial forest lands to the west and north in various stages of harvest, replant, and growth. Imagine how different the scene must have looked when the Indians called this land their home. The trail now switchbacks down through oak savanna, which is undergoing habitat restoration. If there are small flags in the meadows please respect them as they are for research plots. View the picnic shelter below. Just past the last switchback notice the massive oak; the encroaching Douglas-firs have been thinned away, giving the stately tree a chance at living for another hundred years. Return to the shady woods and complete the loop.

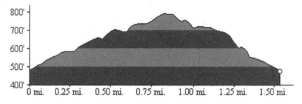

Created with TOPO!® National Geographic

Trail 42. Fort Hoskins Interpretive Trail

Length: 0.6-mile loop • Elevation gain: 85 feet
Difficulty: Easy • Trail uses: Foot, bike, horse
Trail surface: Gravel
Seasonal closures: Open year round
Management agency: Benton County

A full appreciation of the historical aspects of the park is only possible with a walk of the 0.6 mile interpretive trail. There are eight interpretive displays that tell the story of the Indians, the military fort, the Frantz house, the Hoskins school, the early Kings Valley community, and the railroad. The trail starts at the picnic shelter and loops around the former "parade ground" of the Fort. It is a short, yet pleasant and interesting stroll.

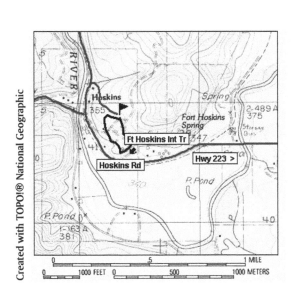

Dunn Forest

North of McDonald Forest lays the 4,030-acre Dunn Forest, also managed by the OSU College of Forestry. There are no trails built for recreation use on the Dunn Forest but there are many miles of gravel roads and year round they can accommodate equestrians, mountain bikers, and those on foot.

What is now the Dunn Forest was once part of the Camp Adair Military Reservation where over 60,000 troops trained during World War II. This tract of land was acquired in 1947 through the efforts of School of Forestry Dean Paul M. Dunn.

As described in the 2005 McDonald-Dunn Forest Management Plan, the Dunn Forest is primarily managed as Theme 1 and Theme 2. Theme 1 areas maximize yield of Douglas-fir on short rotations, thirty-five to forty-five years. These plantations are financially competitive with intensively managed forest plantations worldwide. They are the leading edge in the forest industry for western Oregon. Grasses, herbs, woody shrubs, and hardwoods are viewed as competing vegetation and are generally removed. The southern portion of the Dunn Forest is managed as Theme 1. There are, however, a few scattered parcels of old-growth reserve in the southern portion, with trees over 160 years old.

Theme 2 lands are also even-aged Douglas-fir plantations managed to optimize yield of high-quality wood, but the rotation on these lands is sixty to ninety years. Vegetation management is similar to Theme 1 for the first two to three years after planting but the understory is then allowed to recover. Commercial thinning can occur periodically in both Theme 1 and Theme 2 parcels. The northern portion of the Dunn Forest is managed as Theme 2.

On both Theme 1 and Theme 2 lands recreation is allowed where and when it is compatible. Timber harvesting and limited-access, walk-in hunting are two activities that may restrict recreation use. Recreationists should call the College of Forestry recorded message at 737-4434 to learn of current restrictions and should also check the information kiosks at the trailheads for current information.

While the Dunn Forest may not be as attractive or as accommodating to recreationists as the McDonald Forest, it does have its merits. It is generally quiet with far fewer people. It offers good views. The many miles of forest roads are open year round and are a viable alternative, especially for horses and mountain bikes during the winter when many area trails are seasonally closed. It is not far from Corvallis and offers yet another place to explore

Note: As mentioned, the Dunn Forest is managed primarily for timber production. The forest I describe may be harvested in the future, and current harvest sites will be replanted and new forest will grow.

To get there: There are two ways to reach the access points into Dunn Forest. The most direct way from Corvallis is to drive 6 miles north from Walnut Blvd. on Hwy. 99. Turn left on Tampico Rd. The Rd. 400 gate and information kiosk is in 2.5 miles, on the left, across from Andrews Lane. The pullout has room for just a few cars The Rd. 100 gate is another 2.5 miles further, also on the left, or 5 miles from Hwy. 99 on Tampico Rd.

A curvier but more scenic approach is to follow the directions to the Lewisburg Saddle entrance of McDonald Forest: from Walnut Blvd., travel north on Highland for 2.5 miles, left on Lewisburg Rd, veer right on Sulphur Springs Rd. to the saddle. Continue over the saddle 1 mile. Turn right on Soap Creek Rd. and follow it 4.9 miles east to a "T" with Tampico Rd. Turn left on Tampico. The Rd. 400 gate is in 1.2 miles. The Rd. 100 gate is 2.5 miles further.

Trail 43. Soap Creek Loop

Length: 6.4-mile loop • **Elevation gain:** 1,150 feet
Difficulty: Moderate • **Trail uses:** Foot, bike, horse
Trail surface: Gravel
Seasonal closures: Open year round
Management agency: OSU College of Forestry

On a clear day this loop offers views in all directions, including an excellent view of the Cascades to the east, and Soap Creek Valley and the ridgeline from Peavy Arboretum to Dimple Hill to the south. It passes through or looks upon a variety of areas, from fresh harvest sites to fairly recent replanted forest plantation to attractive second-growth forest, and even an ecologically diverse old-growth parcel. On a day with fog or low clouds the far-ranging views are obscured, but the fog softens the edges of the harvest areas making it still an attractive and interesting loop. The loop can be done in either direction; I describe it counter-clockwise.

This trail starts from the Rd. 400 gate. From the gate, Rd. 400 climbs moderately for a short distance to a junction with Rd. 420. Turn right on Rd. 420. The road is fairly level for a short while then starts to climb up the north side of a hill. On the second of two switchbacks there is a good spot to look across the Willamette Valley. Top out on a ridge with views to the north and south through the trees. Directly in front of you to the west is a pyramid-shaped peak referred to as Old Forest Peak. (This trail description has a side trip option to scramble up the south side of this peak.) Rd. 420 drops down along the ridge then resumes climbing moderately. Turn left at the junction with Rd. 300 and continue traveling up and along the base of Old Forest Peak. You will come to a three-way junction.

To make the side trip up to the grassy meadow on the peak, find the faint path just a few paces back that angles back to the northeast. Follow this path steeply up as it becomes overgrown and almost nonexistent. Cross an old road and keep heading up and you will come out into the meadows. Retrace your steps back down to the junction.

To continue the loop veer left at the previous three-way junction, and then left again onto Rd. 400. The level area

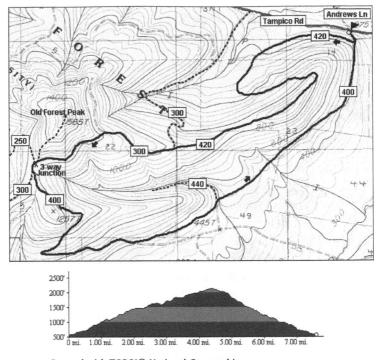

Created with TOPO!® National Geographic

through here is designated old-growth reserve and is lovely to pass through. As the road emerges from the trees above a rock quarry there is a good view all around, including a view of the Cascades from Mt. Hood to Mt. Bachelor. The road descends and heads east along the north side of Soap Creek Valley and passes along the edge of OSU's College of Agriculture Soap Creek Ranch.

At mile 5 there is an abandoned road (Rd. 440) gated to vehicles that also makes a nice side-trip. This soft mossy and overgrown road gently climbs along the side of a creek in a narrow and lush little valley of towering maples. It is worth following it up for a short ways, especially in the spring when there is a good display of wildflowers.

Follow Rd. 400 back to the first junction to complete the loop and then on down to the trailhead.

Trail 44. Berry Creek Loop

Length: 6.3-mile loop • **Elevation gain:** 750 feet
Difficulty: Moderate • **Trail uses:** Foot, bike, horse
Trail surface: Gravel
Seasonal closures: Open year round
Management agency: OSU College of Forestry

This loop, which starts from the Rd. 100 gate, gains less elevation than the Soap Creek Loop. The trail going both to and from the actual loop crosses the pleasing north fork of Berry Creek. The large open harvested areas are stark but provide far-reaching views to the east.

From the orange gate, head southwest on Rd. 100, climbing gradually through open fields managed by OSU College of Agriculture. Staying on Rd. 100, make a sharp turn to the right where Rds. 150 and 170 continue straight ahead. Rd. 100 then curves and crosses over Berry Creek and then splits at the next junction to make a loop. Turn left on Rd. 100 and a short ways later make a sharp left up-hill on Rd. 190. Climb along the edge of a harvest with forest to the west and an open view to the

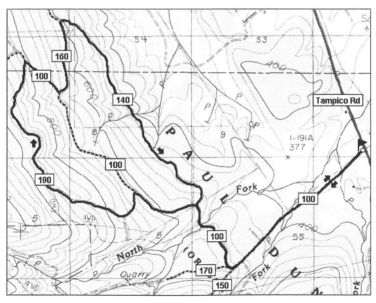

Created with TOPO!® National Geographic

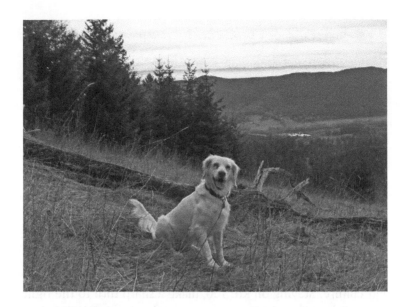

east. Re-enter the woods and come to a junction with Rd. 100. Turn right, and in 0.5 mile turn left on Rd. 160. In another 0.5 mile, turn right on Rd. 140 and follow it back to its junction with Rd. 100, where the loop started. Turn left, cross Berry Creek again, and follow Rd. 100 back to the gate.

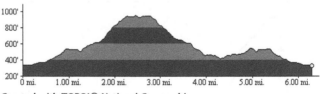

Created with TOPO!® National Geographic

Baskett Slough
National Wildlife Refuge

Oregon has a number of National Wildlife Refuges that help protect many wildlife species as well as preserving the diverse habitats that support them. Three of these refuges are in the Willamette Valley and are within an hour's drive from Corvallis. Baskett Slough, Ankeny, and William Finley National Wildlife Refuges were all created in the 1960s and their primary goal is to provide wintering habitat for dusky Canada Geese. "Duskies" nest exclusively on the Copper River Delta in Alaska and winter almost solely in the Willamette Valley. In the winter there are literally thousands of them, along with other waterfowl, and at Baskett Slough you can observe them from a viewpoint right off Hwy. 22, from inside your car on the road through the refuge, or, best of all, from the top of easily ascended Baskett Butte.

Like the other refuges, Baskett Slough provides a wonderful opportunity for an outing to observe wildlife, get some exercise, and appreciate some historic habitat of the Willamette Valley. At 2,492 acres, Baskett Slough was established in 1964 and named for George J. Baskett, an early Willamette Valley thoroughbred-horse breeder. With a mixture of shallow marshes and ponds, gentle oak savannah hills, and farmed fields, Baskett Slough is lovely and brimming with life.

Perhaps as an unexpected consequence of this area's having been preserved over forty years ago, Baskett Slough is now also home to one of the last and largest remnant populations of the Fender's Blue butterfly. Thought to be extinct for several decades, they were rediscovered in 1989. A close association was observed between the butterflies and Kincaid's lupine, which is the primary food source for the butterflies during their larval stage. The native upland prairie and oak savannah of Baskett Butte contain an abundance of lupine and, provided with federal protection in 2000, these two species will be able to flourish. The adult butterflies emerge in May and June and visiting at this time will likely yield glimpses of these beautiful little butterflies. The refuge hosts a Fender's Blue Butterfly Day on the Butte in mid-May.

There is a viewpoint on Hwy. 22 that overlooks the southern half of the refuge and the large marshes where the dusky geese winter. Coville Rd. passes east-west through the refuge, connecting Hwys. 22 and 99, providing a more close-up view of the marshes and waterfowl. Bring your binoculars and a picnic.

To get there: From Walnut Blvd. in Corvallis, travel north on Hwy. 99 for 24 miles. Cross Hwy. 22 and drive north 2 more miles. Turn left on Coville Rd. to reach the Baskett Butte trailhead. One mile beyond Coville Rd. on Hwy. 99, turn left on Smithfield Rd. for 2.5 miles to reach Morgan Lake and Moffitti Marsh trailhead.

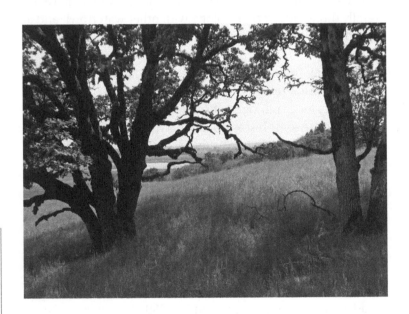

Trail 45. Baskett Butte Observation Platform and Loop Trail

Length: 1.4-mile loop • Elevation gain: 160 feet
Difficulty: Easy • Trail uses: Foot
Trail surface: Gravel, mowed grass
Seasonal closures: Open year round
Managing agency: U.S. Fish and Wildlife Service
Other information: Dogs not allowed. No hunting

Baskett Butte Observation Platform and Loop Trail afford the opportunity to walk up through attractive native oak savannah, enjoy the view overlooking the bucolic Willamette Valley countryside, and observe birds and waterfowl. The platform and trail are situated right in the middle of the refuge, and access is from a trailhead on Coville Rd. The trail climbs moderately for 0.75 mile on a wide sand and gravel path through open oak prairie that is slowly being restored to its native character. At the first junction, keep left; the loop will finish on the trail to the right. This is the area that is home to the many Kincaid's lupines and Fender's Blue butterflies. From the platform on Baskett Butte, formerly called Mt. Baldy, look south, east, and west at the rolling hills of the valley, the mosaic of farms and vineyards, and some large, vital marshes in the

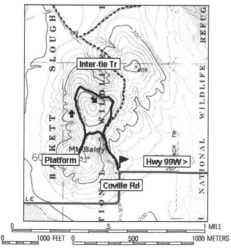

Created with TOPO!® National Geographic

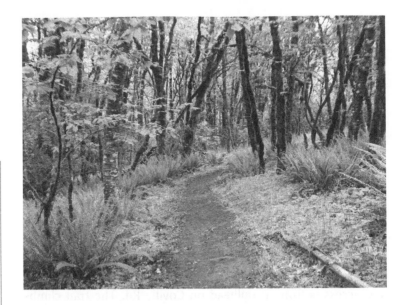

refuge. The hearty honking of the geese and other waterfowl can be quite entertaining.

To add the 1-mile loop, go back to the last junction and take the mowed grass path that heads north. Soon you will enter lovely oak woodlands lush with sword ferns as the trail curves along the north side of the butte. In spring the floor is a carpet of small pink geraniums. The music of songbirds fills the air. At a mowed grass junction on the east side, turn right to complete the loop past some magnificent white oaks and return to the trailhead.

Or, if it is a good day for walking and you want to do another 3.7 miles, turn left at the previous junction and take the 0.6 mile Inter-tie Trail north and loop around Morgan Lake and Moffitti Marsh (see Trail 46). These trails are open April 1st through Sept 30th and offer some nice marsh-life viewing.

Trail 46. Morgan Lake and Moffitti Marsh Loop Trail

Length: 2.5-mile loop • **Elevation gain**: 70 feet
Difficulty: Easy to moderate • **Trail uses**: Foot
Trail surface: Gravel, mowed grass
Seasonal closures: Closed 10/1 to 3/31
Managing agency: U.S. Fish and Wildlife Service
Other information: Dogs not allowed. No hunting or
fishing

The trailhead is across Smithfield Rd. from an old barn on the right. Most of this trail is out in the open and is not suggested for midday in summer. As with most loops, it can be done in either direction. I describe it clockwise. Walk south on the gravel path, up a short, gentle grade and you will be on the bank of Morgan Lake. From here there is a wide view of the idyllic north side of the refuge and surrounding hills and farms. Look for geese, mallards, teals, red-winged blackbirds, and marsh wrens. As you leave the lake and continue south towards Baskett Butte you will walk around a farmed field and up a pretty good climb, then down the other side to a junction. Left takes you up to Baskett Butte; right continues the loop. Moffitti Marsh is delightful and just bursting with bird life. Follow the road around the marsh. At Smithfield Rd. there is a mowed grass path to take you back to the trailhead.

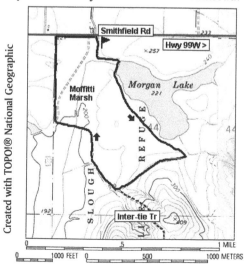

Ankeny National Wildlife Refuge

Ankeny National Wildlife Refuge, like the others in the Willamette Valley, offers dusky Canada geese the three things that they need to prepare them for their migration in the spring: food, water, and sanctuary. The cultivated farm fields within the refuge provide nutritious, high-protein grasses. A cooperative agreement with the U.S. Fish and Wildlife Service and the farmers works well; the farmers plant rye and other grasses in the late summer that is ready for the fall arrival of the geese. After they leave in the spring, the farmer harvests the grass seed. The refuge provides water in the form of wetlands, either natural or restored by the U.S. Fish and Wildlife Service. Sanctuary is provided in the 2,796 acres of flat to gently rolling fields, hedgerows, Oregon ash forests, and wetlands where the geese and other waterfowl can rest undisturbed while they regain energy for their spring migrations. Like all the wildlife refuges, a visit to Ankeny is quite peaceful, though the refuge is just a couple of miles from the noisy I-5 corridor.

Ankeny is home to numerous other wildlife species as well, including a multitude of waterfowl like wood ducks, grebes, herons, and easy-to-spot tall, white egrets. Soaring above the marshes are bald eagles, osprey, hawks, and falcons. During spring the refuge is a chorus of songbirds. Red fox and black-tailed deer also inhabit the refuge. There are a few boardwalks and viewing platforms where visitors with binoculars can easily view many of the above species. Ankeny Overlook, on the north end of the refuge on Ankeny Hill Rd., looks out over the entire refuge, provides general information, and has public restrooms. Eagle Marsh Kiosk on the west side of the refuge, on Buena Vista Rd., provides excellent opportunities for viewing wildlife activity on the biggest marsh on Ankeny. The Pintail and Egret Marsh Boardwalk, off Wintel Rd., leads visitors through a short, wooded slough to an observation blind where they can spy on bustling marsh wildlife. The Rail Trail Boardwalk and Observation Blind, also off Wintel Rd., offer a little longer stroll through a wetland forest to an observation blind overlooking Wood Duck Pond.

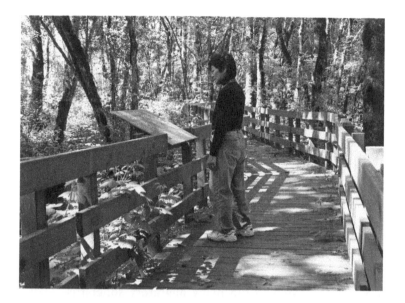

The above boardwalks and viewing platforms are open year round. Bring your binoculars.

To get there: From Albany, drive 10 miles north on I-5 to exit 243, Ankeny Hill Rd. Drive west 0.25 mile to an intersection of Ankeny Hill Rd. and Wintel Rd. If you have the time for a 7-mile driving loop preview around the refuge with stops at the viewing kiosks and observation decks before walking the Rail Trail Loop you will have a much fuller appreciation of the refuge. In this case turn right on Ankeny Hill Rd. In 2.3 miles turn left on Buena Vista Rd. and left again in 2.8 miles on Wintel Rd. It is 1.8 miles to the Rail Trail trailhead on the right. If you are not driving around the refuge then turn left on Wintel Rd. at the Ankeny/Wintel junction and travel 2 miles to the trailhead on the left.

Trail 47. Rail Trail Loop

Length: 2-mile loop • **Elevation gain:** 15 feet
Difficulty: Easy • **Trail uses:** Foot
Trail surface: Wooden boardwalk, mowed grass, gravel
Seasonal closures: Boardwalk to blind open year
   round; Rail Trail beyond closed 10/1 to 3/31
Management agency: U.S. Fish and Wildlife Service
Other information: Dogs not allowed. No hunting or
   fishing

The level path heads south from the parking area through a lovely Oregon ash wetland. Turn right 0.25 mile in on the enchanting and curving boardwalk. This wetland floods in the winter and dries up during the summer. During spring and fall look for and listen to the many migratory songbirds. Native wildflowers are abundant in the spring. There are interpretive signs along the way. The year-round boardwalk ends at the observation blind on Wood Duck Pond. The pond is full and bustling with life during winter and spring, but is nearly dry by late summer. The seasonally open boardwalk continues to wrap around the pond, then ends on a dike. Cross the dike and follow the simple trail through shaded forest before coming back up onto the dike. Turn right and walk along the wide, grassy dike back to the boardwalk junction. Return on the boardwalk, or for a longer walk, continue along the dike around Dunlin Pond, also vibrant with pond life in spring but

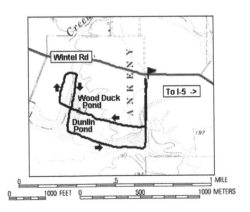

Created with TOPO!® National Geographic

nearly dry by late summer. Under the midday sun, this section can be quite warm, but it is nice in early morning or evening. At the first fork on the south side of the pond, veer left, then left again on the mowed path just a few yards further. These forks are unsigned, but will connect you back to the main trail right where the boardwalk began. Follow the shady corridor back to the parking area.

Takena Landing Park

Takena Landing Park is a 72-acre Albany City park on the north bank of the Willamette River. There is a boat landing, as well as picnic tables, restrooms, and a trail along the river.

To get there: From the east side of Corvallis, where Circle Blvd. ends at Hwy. 20, drive 7.9 miles northeast on Hwy. 20. Turn right at the stoplight on North Albany Rd., before crossing the bridge into Albany. This road ends in 0.2 miles at Takena Landing Park. The trail starts under the highway bridge.

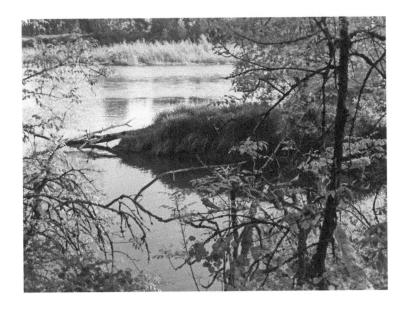

Trail 48. Takena Landing Trail

Length: 4 miles round trip • Elevation gain:
   insignificant
Difficulty: Easy • Trail uses: Foot, bike
Trail surface: Packed earth, muddy in rainy weather
Seasonal closures: Open year round
Managing agency: Albany City Parks

This short and level trail hugs close to the Willamette River and provides an easy walk through a nice riparian corridor. The towering cottonwoods are impressive and the masses of vines climbing up and draping over the branches are unusual. The path is packed dirt so this trail is best when dry. Winter conditions will be muddy, and during heavy rains when the river is high, the trail may be under water. Spring, summer, and fall are the time for a walk here. Trail construction is an ongoing Eagle Scout project.

The trail starts directly under the highway bridge. The traffic noise lessens as you get further along the trail. The first part of the trail parallels the Golf Club of Oregon. Pass under the railroad trestle and continue along the river. There are intermittent views of the river through the shrubbery. The trail makes a short loop at the end before coming back.

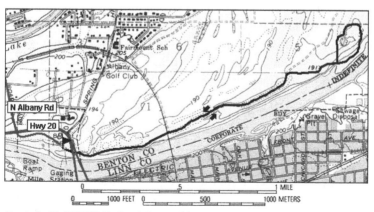

Created with TOPO!® National Geographic

McDowell Creek Falls Park

Just 33 miles from Corvallis, tucked in a valley north of Sweet Home, lies a hidden jewel in the foothills of the Cascades. Set in a deep, lush glen, this Linn County park has two impressive waterfalls, other smaller falls, deep pools, a misty grotto loaded with dripping moss and ferns, and an easy, well-maintained trail with sturdy bridges to view it all from. It is a great hike for children as there is lots of "wow" within a short distance. It can also provide anyone with impressive waterfall photos. The spring wildflowers are beautiful and the fall maple color is terrific. Parents who have taken their kids to Camp Tadmore may not realize what a lush and lovely environment lies on either side of the road leading into the camp. It is worth exploring. The park is named for Jack McDowell, an early settler in the area.

There are at least three ways to visit the waterfalls in this park. The first option has just a slight elevation gain and is an out-and-back on the main trail for a 1.5-mile round trip that stays along the creek the entire way. Since there is also a high trail, you can also make a loop, though this involves a short section of road walking. This loop, also 1.5 miles in length, can be done in either direction, depending on whether you are more comfortable going up or down a very steep set of 140 stairs. The following trail description and elevation profile makes the loop in the counterclockwise direction, climbing the steep stairs early in the hike and then returning by following the gentle trail downstream.

To get there: To reach McDowell Creek Falls Park, drive 24.5 miles east of Corvallis on Hwy. 20, or 4.4 miles east of the last light in Lebanon. Turn left at the brown sign for McDowell Creek Falls and follow the signs for 9 paved miles as you head north through pleasant rolling hills, gradually gaining elevation. There are three parking areas; I recommend stopping at the first and walking the length of the park. There is a restroom at this lower lot and picnic tables around all three parking areas. Some of the tables are draped in a tablecloth of moss. Do not leave valuables in your car.

Trail 49. McDowell Creek Falls Loop

Length: 1.5-mile loop • **Elevation gain:** 310 feet
Difficulty: Moderate • **Trail uses:** Foot
Trail surface: Packed earth, gravel, wooden boardwalk
Seasonal closures: Open year round
Managing agency: Linn County

As soon as you exit your car you are greeted by the sound of McDowell Creek, be it roaring or burbling. Whether you are doing an out-and-back along the creek or a loop, the trail starts at the end of the parking lot and immediately crosses McDowell Creek on the first of several well-built bridges. The trail winds along the creek through thick undergrowth of spring flowers and summer berries. Douglas-fir, alder, and maple arch over the trail. Side paths lead to the creek. The trail takes a sharp turn and climbs more steeply. At 0.2 mile the main park trail turns left and crosses the bridge over Fall Creek, where you have a fantastic view of Royal Terrace Falls. This 119-foot waterfall drops over the valley wall in a stair-step or terraced fashion. The main trail, for an out-and-back outing, continues up the lush, narrowing valley, ending on the boardwalk overlooking Majestic Falls. Both falls carry far less water by late summer.

If you are making the loop, however, continue up Fall Creek on the approximately 140 stone steps to the top of Royal Terrace Falls. This gives you a nice view of the smaller upper falls and the secluded pool it drops into, before pouring down the taller section of the falls. The trail then crosses Fall Creek and continues gradually climbing, parallel to the main trail but

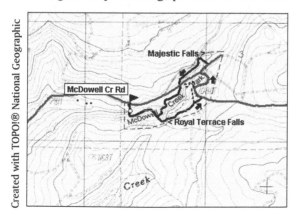

Created with TOPO!® National Geographic

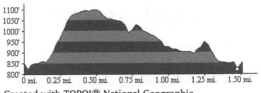

Created with TOPO!® National Geographic

at a higher elevation. This is a classic temperate rain forest consisting of large cedars and maples with moss hanging from the branches. Oxalis, maidenhair ferns, vanilla leaf, and many others comprise the forest floor. The trail crests and begins its route downward.

Cross a bridge over a shallow brook with an abundance of skunk cabbage. At a junction, the left trail heads down somewhat steeply, then switchbacks to the main road just above the bridge over McDowell Creek. Instead, stay to the right and you will soon come to the road. Walk to the left along the road, facing the oncoming traffic, using caution, as the road leads to the popular camp. Walk down the road 0.25 mile, around a curve, and then take the right fork of the road to the upper parking lot and picnic area. Hold on as you descend a creative series of wooden staircases, bridges, and observation decks that can be quite slippery. They take you down into the misty, green grotto of Majestic Falls, an impressive 34-foot curtain-type falls, and the largest falls on McDowell Creek. After getting your fill of this wondrous place, follow the trail down along McDowell Creek through its mossy-walled gulch. Huge cedar stumps attest to past logging activity. Large maples wearing blankets of moss overhang the trail and small rivulets trickle across to join the main creek. The trail then leaves the deepest part of the valley and crosses the main road. Continue following the creek down, pass a junction coming in from the middle parking area and cross over McDowell Creek on a handsome arched bridge. A little further and you will find yourself back on the bridge looking at Royal Terrace Falls once again. Return to the parking area on the trail you started on.

Snag Boat Bend

This as yet little-known piece of property located off Peoria Road on a broad bend in the Willamette River is excellent for bird watching, walking, and nature study. The 341 acres of biologically diverse land is managed by Finley Wildlife Refuge. The Nature Conservancy bought the property from a private landowner in 1998 and transferred it to the U.S. Fish and Wildlife Service in 2000. The Greenbelt Land Trust helped with trail building and habitat restoration, including planting over six thousand native trees. The property opened to the public in 2003. Snag Boat Bend represents yet another example of public agencies partnering with private , nonprofit organizations to protect and restore high-quality habitat in the Willamette Valley for wildlife and native plants.

The car traveler on Peoria Road sees miles and miles of richly fertile farmland including 200 acres of Snag Boat Bend that continue to be farmed cooperatively, with the remains after harvest providing browse for wintering geese. What is hidden from the road and awaiting quiet observation on foot is the attractive floodplain forest, vital marshes, and lush backwater sloughs of the Willamette River with its inhabitants of great blue herons, ospreys, bald eagles, hawks, songbirds, western

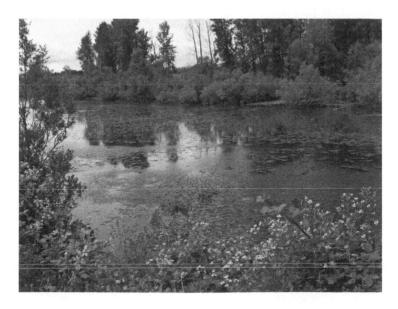

pond turtles, red-legged frogs, and the thousands of visiting waterfowl in the fall, winter, and spring. Bring your binoculars.

Like the other wildlife refuges in the valley, there are some restrictions for public access. The refuge is open from sunrise to sunset. Bicycles, horses, and dogs are prohibited. Only the short boardwalk to the observation platform is open year round. Trails beyond the boardwalk are closed from October 1 through January 31; hunting and fishing is allowed during that time by boat access. Check with U.S. Fish and Wildlife Service.

To date there are 1.25 miles of trail here, but walks of a few miles can easily be accomplished. Future plans include an additional few miles of trail along the Willamette River and its sloughs that will take the visitor through superb riparian habitat.

To get there: From Corvallis, cross the Van Buren bridge and travel 1 mile east on Hwy. 34. Turn right on Peoria Rd. Snag Boat Bend is on the right in 10.8 miles, just past Oxbow Orchard.

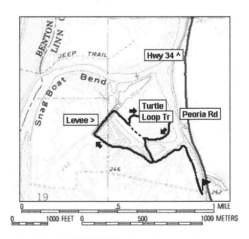

Created with TOPO!® National Geographic

Trail 50. Snag Boat Bend Loop

Length: 2.1-mile loop • Elevation gain: insignificant
Difficulty: Easy • Trail uses: Foot
Trail surface: Wooden boardwalk, mowed grass,
   packed earth, gravel
Seasonal closures: Closed beyond platform at 0.07
   miles 10/1 to 1/31
Managing agency: U.S. Fish and Wildlife Service

From the parking area, follow the wooden boardwalk a short 0.07 mile to the observation platform overlooking the beaver pond. Here the trail becomes a mowed path lined with blackberry bushes. In 0.25 mile, there is a picnic table, which is a good place to look for western pond turtles in the quiet backwater. In another 0.25 mile, there is a junction with the Turtle Loop Trail on the right. Continue straight and you will see the junction to the observation blind, an octagonal wooden structure with viewing windows to discreetly observe wildlife on the backwater slough. After leaving the observation blind, continue west along the farmed fields and turn right at the next junction. Walk along the raised levee overlooking the Willamette River for 0.25 mile, keeping an eye out for heron and osprey. Turn right and drop down into the lower floodplain forest of the Turtle Loop Trail. Shortly, the trail splits to make the loop. Turn left and follow the trail through large cottonwoods along the backwater slough of Lake Creek. At the next junction, turn left through a very wet area that may be flooded during winter and spring, but is excellent habitat for rearing salmon and pond turtles as well as many species of shorebirds. (If it is too wet to get through here, continue on the Turtle Loop back to the levee and retrace your route out the way you came.) Return to the main trail near the observation blind. Turn left one more time and follow the trail back in.

William L. Finley
National Wildlife Refuge

If you are not familiar with Finley Wildlife Refuge, less than 10 miles south of Corvallis, then you should make a point of becoming acquainted with this truly remarkable place. This 5,325-acre sanctuary protects many historic habitats of the Willamette Valley and provides a safe haven for large and diverse populations of waterfowl and mammals. Many ponds, marshes, and streams are scattered amongst oak savannah, native prairie, bottomland ash forest, maple, second-growth Douglas-fir forests, and wildlife crop fields. Finley is the largest remaining wetland in the valley and thus has an extensive population of native plants. Some of the more recognizable wildflowers include Oregon iris, larkspur, camas, lupine, monkey flower and meadow checker-mallow.

Like the other wildlife refuges in the Willamette Valley, this sanctuary was established to protect the winter habitat of dusky Canada geese and other wintering waterfowl and there are literally thousands of them here during this time. In the spring and fall many species of migratory birds will rest here while on their travels. The ponds and marshes, small and large, are alive with birdsong and a walk along them is refreshing for anyone and a paradise for bird watchers. Finley is also home to a growing herd of Roosevelt elk; one fresh and misty day in April, my daughter and I had the good fortune to observe nearly one hundred elk as we walked up Pigeon Butte. Other mammals that call Finley home include beaver, ground squirrels, black-tailed deer, and black bear.

Established in 1964, Finley is the largest and most southern of three wildlife refuges in the Willamette Valley managed by the U.S. Fish and Wildlife Service. William Finley made major contributions to wildlife conservation in Oregon and persuaded President Theodore Roosevelt to establish the first wildlife refuges west of the Mississippi. Early settler history from the Applegate Trail can be observed at the small 1855 John Feichter house just off the main refuge road.

Wildlife Refuge Rd. and Bruce Rd. both traverse east-west through the refuge and are open all year, dawn till dusk.

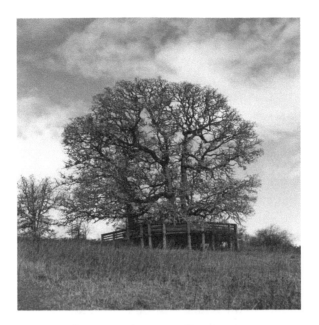

The trails are for foot traffic only; no bikes or horses. Dogs are not allowed on any of the trails at any time; they may only be let out of vehicles at kiosks or trailhead parking areas and then must be on a leash. Bikes are allowed on Wildlife Refuge Rd. and Bruce Rd. only between April 1st and October 31, when just about all of the refuge is open; the interior service roads are considered trails, and bikes cannot be ridden on them at any time. Between November 1st and March 31st, all but the western quarter of the refuge is closed to recreation. This is a time to observe the geese, other waterfowl, and perhaps even the elk herd from your car or at viewpoints, and walk Woodpecker Loop or the Mill Hill trails.

Bring your binoculars. To accompany this guide, there are maps available at all the roadside kiosks.

To get there: To access Finley NWR from the east side, travel Hwy. 99W 8.5 miles south from Avery Ave./Crystal Lake Dr. and turn right on Wildlife Refuge Rd. To reach the more southern road through the refuge continue 2.7 miles further south and turn right on Bruce Rd.

To access Finley from the west side, travel south on 53rd St, turn right on Plymouth Rd. in Philomath, and continue south on Bellfountain Rd. for 9.3 miles. Turn left at Wildlife Refuge Rd. or continue another 3.2 miles and turn left on Bruce Rd.

Trail 51. Woodpecker Loop

Length: 1-mile loop • **Elevation gain:** 130 feet
Difficulty: Easy • **Trail uses:** Foot
Trail surface: Gravel, wooden boardwalk
Seasonal closures: Open year round
Managing agency: U.S. Fish and Wildlife Service
Other information: No dogs

Woodpecker Loop is the most popular trail at Finley NWR. Designated in 2005 as a National Recreation Trail, one of only four in Oregon, Woodpecker Loop gives visitors an exposure to various habitats as well as an overlook of the refuge, the Willamette Valley, and the Coast Range. This lightly graveled trail with sturdy bridges and boardwalk over marshy areas makes for good wet-season walking. The trailhead is near the west entrance of the refuge, just off Refuge Rd.

Just a few hundred feet in, the trail forks to make the loop. Walking in either direction is fine, though I prefer left, clockwise. Travel through maple forest, then low-lying ash, and Douglas-fir, and past a couple of ponds. Read the interpretive signs describing the various birds (woodpeckers in particular) and other animals that live in these habitats. Top out in oak savannah and from the viewing platform under the huge white oak you can look out on acres of this native oak prairie, including Bald Top to the northeast. For a longer hike, take the 0.5-mile Inter-Tie connector trail and add in the 3-mile Mill Hill Loop (Trail 52) to your outing.

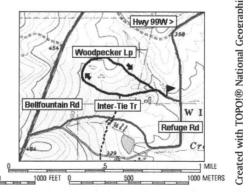

Trail 52. Mill Hill Loop

Length: 3.1-mile loop • Elevation gain: 220 feet
Difficulty: Easy • Trail uses: Foot
Trail surface: Mowed grass, gravel, packed earth
Seasonal closures: Open year round
Managing agency: U.S. Fish and Wildlife Service
Other information: No dogs

The Mill Hill Loop is open year round, but in the winter it is a good deal muddier than the Woodpecker Loop and wearing boots is advised. The trail begins at the Display Pond parking area and kiosk at the west end of Refuge Rd.

From the information sign walk west along the fence on a mowed grass path. The trail turns south and the Inter-Tie trail connects in from Woodpecker Loop. The trail follows along the gravel service road for a few hundred yards to a junction. In the winter, the servicce road to the left is closed; the loop begins just a bit further to the right. Follow the loop in either direction. The trail travels gently up and down through various forest types. The most interesting area is along the Gray Creek swamp, where some wildlife may be spotted. For a longer walk from April through October, take the above-mentioned service road on to Beaver and Cattail Pond Loop (Trail 54) or, further yet, to Cabell Marsh (Trail 53).

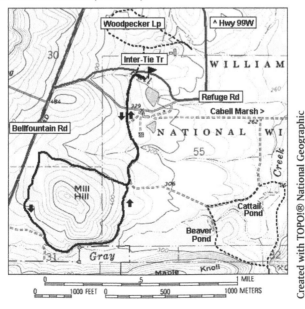

Created with TOPO!® National Geographic

Trail 53. Cabell Marsh Trail

Length: 2 miles round trip • **Elevation gain:** 50 feet
Difficulty: Easy • **Trail uses:** Foot
Trail surface: Gravel
Seasonal closures: Closed 11/1 to 3/31
Managing agency: U.S. Fish and Wildlife Service
Other information: No dogs

This waterfowl viewing area is just bursting with life. Though fairly short by itself on an out-and-back path, it can be a wonderful start and finish for a longer water-habitat hike with Beaver and Cattail Ponds (Trail 54) or up onto Pigeon Butte (Trail 55) for a fine view of the valley to the south. Future plans call for a trail along the west side of the marsh, which will make for an exquisite loop. The trail begins at the refuge headquarters parking area in the middle of the refuge, just south of Refuge Rd.

Walk the brief distance to the attractive viewing and interpretive kiosk. Follow the short path to the service road and turn right. You are walking along a human-made dike that backs up flowing waters to create this large marsh. Keep your

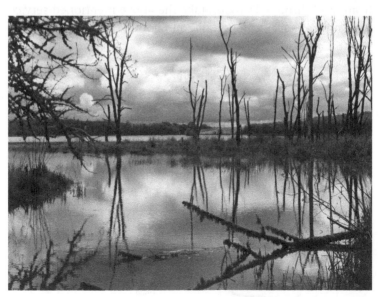

William L. Finley National Wildlife Refuge • Cabell Marsh Trail

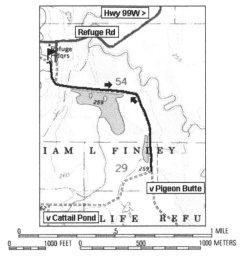

Created with TOPO!® National Geographic

eyes and ears open for great blue herons, osprey, wood ducks, and a melody of song birds. In April you may see and hear geese still preparing for their journey north and in October witness the first arrivals back to Finley. Summer evenings are exceptionally nice. The trail turns back at the signed junction. To continue on to Pigeon Butte from here, follow the service road south. Or to add in Cattail and Beaver Pond Loop, turn right and continue west on a service road along the edge of the marsh until you come to Cattail Pond.

Trail 54. Beaver and Cattail Pond Loop

Length: 2.3-mile loop • **Elevation gain:** 15 feet
Difficulty: Easy • **Trail uses:** Foot
Trail surface: Mowed grass, packed earth, gravel
Seasonal closures: Closed 11/1 to 3/31
Managing agency: U.S. Fish and Wildlife Service
Other information: No dogs

This pond and marsh habitat loop is delightful and easy by itself and also works well combined with the Mill Hill Loop or Cabell Marsh Trail for a longer hike. There is good opportunity for observing pond inhabitants such as beaver, ducks, and migrating birds. Brilliant red-winged blackbirds dwell in these cattail marshes and dragonflies hover above the ponds. There is also an impressive collection of lowland spring wildflowers and blooming pink spirea in the summer. Unlike at Jackson-Frazier Wetland with its raised boardwalk, you will get your feet wet here, so wear boots and enjoy it.

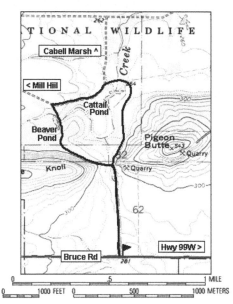

Created with TOPO!® National Geographic

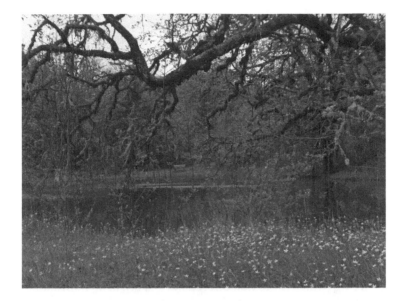

There is a signed parking area near the west end of the refuge on the north side of Bruce Rd. The trail heads straight north on a section of the old Applegate trail that is now a mowed grass path in a tunnel of overhanging trees. The trail forks at the old rock quarry site on the edge of Pigeon Butte. Make the loop in either direction; left visits Beaver Pond first and right visits Cattail Pond first. The service road connects the two, as well as leading west to Mill Hill and north to Cabell Marsh.

Trail 55. Pigeon Butte Trail

Length: 3 miles round trip • **Elevation gain**: 285 feet
Difficulty: Easy • **Trail uses**: Foot
Trail surface: Gravel
Seasonal closures: Closed 11/1 to 3/31
Managing agency: U.S. Fish and Wildlife Service
Other information: No dogs. There is a lot of poison oak.

Pigeon Butte is the highest point in the refuge and allows for terrific views of the Willamette Valley. It is named for the band-tailed pigeons that inhabit the oak woodlands on the top and flanks of the butte. It can be reached on foot from the north via the service road from Cabell Marsh, or as a walk from Bruce Rd (which is the trail offered here). Park at an information overlook on the south side of Bruce Rd., just west of McFadden Marsh (this is a wonderful marsh). Walk across Bruce Rd. and head north on a service road toward the red barn on the hill. At Cheadle Pond veer west and then north again. An unmarked but obvious path leaves the road to the west and climbs easily up through the old quarry and on up to the top. The huge Oregon white oaks up here are beautiful but beware that this is prime poison oak habitat as well. If you're lucky the elk herd will be in the area.

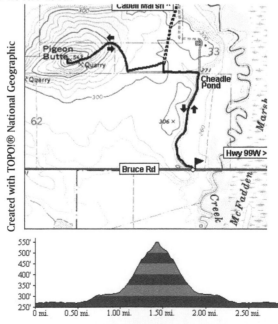

Alsea Falls Recreation Area

Alsea Falls Recreation Site is a perfect example of classic Northwest rain forest with huge Douglas-firs and western red cedars towering over vine maple and a verdant green understory of mosses, ferns, oxalis, exceptional spring wildflowers, and the smooth-flowing Alsea River with its cascading falls. It is a lovely area for heralding in spring in western Oregon. On a hot summer day it is one of the coolest and most refreshing places in Benton County that I know of. This riparian oasis is surrounded by a patchwork of industrial forest lands, which helps one appreciate this gem all the more.

Alsea Falls is a Bureau of Land Management (BLM) recreation site. There are about 4 miles of hiking trails along the river, some of which are open to bikes. Across the road there are close to 10 miles of mountain biking/hiking trails. There are an abundance of nicely situated picnic tables, a restroom, and drinking water in the day use area and a campground with sixteen sites. Both the campground and day use area are open mid-May through September, and they are gated during the remaining months. The bike trail across the road is accessible year round.

To get there: The 30-mile drive from Corvallis is a pleasant tour; the road from Alpine to Alsea is a BLM National Back Country Byway. From South 53rd St in Corvallis, turn right on Plymouth Rd. and travel west to its junction with Belfountain Rd. in Philomath. Turn left on Belfountain Rd. and travel 16 miles south to Alpine. Turn right (west) and follow signs to Alsea Falls for 9 more miles. The day use area is 1 mile past the campground entrance, both on the right. The trailhead for the bike trail is half way between the campground and the day use area on the left, just a short ways in. To make the drive a loop, continue on another 9 miles to Alsea and return to Corvallis on Hwy. 34.

Trail 56. Alsea River Trail

Length: 1-mile loop • **Elevation gain:** 15 feet
Difficulty: Easy • **Trail uses:** Foot, bike
Trail surface: Packed earth
Seasonal closures: Closed 10/1 to 5/15
Managing agency: Bureau of Land Management

The most frequently walked trail here runs between the day use/picnic area and the campground and returns on the other side of the river. This 1-mile loop is nearly level, curves and winds through handsome forest, and is almost entirely in the shade. The trees along here are fairly large and old, but not nearly as old as the huge stumps from harvests as long ago as the 1850s. The BLM has built two graceful arching bridges over the river at either end of this trail, so rock hopping or wading across is no longer necessary. This short loop is also open to bikers, who can continue upriver along the bank for another mile to a gravel road which intersects the Byway.

From the far side of the river there are other options, for foot travel only, to make a longer hike. One is to turn left (north) at the lower bridge and walk down the Alsea River another mile to

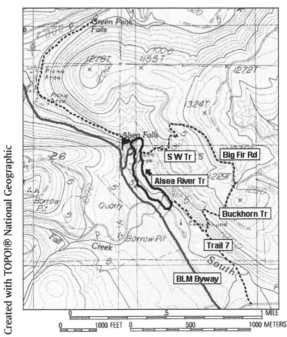

Alsea Falls Recreation Area • Alsea River Trail

Created with TOPO!® National Geographic

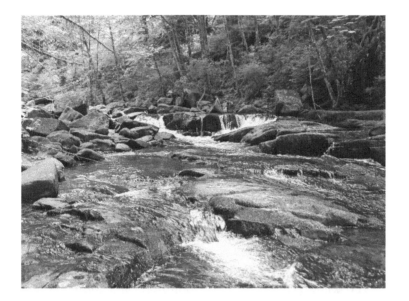

Green Peak Falls on Peak Creek. This allows you to continue the beautiful forest walk along the river and see other charming smaller falls and pools. In 0.5 mile the trail will seem to end on a gravel lane. Follow it to the left and then take the right fork of the gravel road. In just about 50 yards you should see a sign where the trail picks up again on the right and passes around Hubert K. McBee Memorial Park. This is a private park. Follow the trail another 0.5 mile through the cool forest corridor, climb somewhat, and you will hear, and then see, Green Peak Falls, a very lush and inviting setting. Retrace your steps back.

There is another option if you want a short (1.3 miles) but demanding walk. When you cross the upper bridge, turn right on BLM Trail 7. In 0.25 miles turn left on the Buckhorn Trail. This new trail climbs very steeply (up to 20% grade) for 0.45 mile, gaining 400 feet in elevation. Turn left on an old gravel road (Big Fir) and parallel the trail below for 0.5 mile. Turn left at the trail marker and come down 0.4 mile on the equally steep Side Winder Trail.

Trail 57. Alsea Bike Loop

Length: 6-mile loop • **Elevation gain:** 985 feet
Difficulty: Moderate • **Trail uses:** Foot, bike
Trail surface: Paved road, gravel, loosely packed earth
Seasonal closures: Open year round
Managing agency: Bureau of Land Management

This loop is a pleasant trail to walk, but I think it holds even more interest for the mountain biker looking for a challenging ride. It is a combination of gated paved road, gravel road, and newly built but rough single-track trail to connect the road segments. It climbs and descends at a considerable grade and would not be enjoyed by a novice rider. For a fit and more skilled rider it is quite a hoot.

The yellow gate is where the loop starts and finishes. There may or may not be a map posted here. Definitely do the loop counterclockwise; this way the ascent will be on the paved road and the descent will be on gravel and trail. Climb for about 3 miles through shady and attractive forest on a single-lane paved road (Hard Rock) littered with forest debris and branches. The road then levels somewhat and curves around the top end of the loop. Turn left at 3.6 miles on the steep gravel road (Billy Buster) and begin the descent as it alternates between gravel road and rough trails (Bailout and Stellar Jay). Keep an eye out

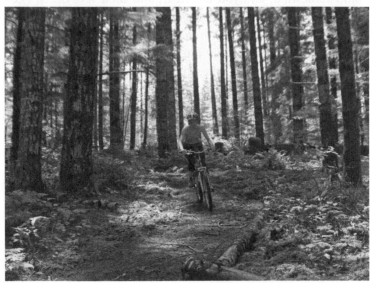

for the brown trail markers. A wrong turn will either lead you to dead-ends or ultimately back down to the Byway via other roads designated for bikes. Assuming you follow the marked but confusing route correctly, the last hundred yards of the Stellar Jay Trail before the gate and parking area is the most attractive as you cross on a sturdy bridge over the exquisite Fall Creek. It is worth a pause here to take in the gentle creek, the enormous ferns and the lush shades of green that exemplify Pacific Northwest forests.

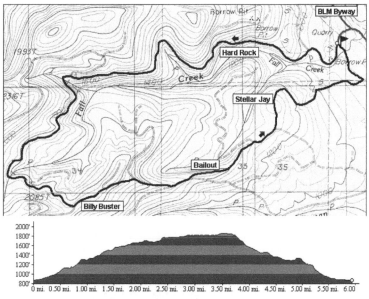

Created with TOPO!® National Geographic

Clemens Park

This small, but quaint, Benton County park along the North Fork of the Alsea River is a popular fishing spot, a good place to watch the salmon run in the fall, and has a lovely walking trail along the river. It is a wonderful place to explore the rich and diverse life of this representative streamside forest of the Oregon Coast Range. Spring brings a carpet of wildflowers to this riparian woodland. Hot summer days in the valley are cooler here; fall is pleasant and colorful, while winter is drippy, but mossy and fresh. There are picnic tables along the river, restrooms, and an information kiosk with interpretive brochures. This park makes a nice picnic-and-a-walk stop while en route to the coast. Rex and Ethel Clemens donated the 37 acres of land for this park to the citizens of Benton County in 1968.

To get there: To reach Clemens Park, drive 14.5 miles on Hwy. 34 from the Hwy. 20/34 split at the west end of Philomath. The park will be on your left, identified by a brown Benton County sign. Clemens Park is 1 mile east of the town of Alsea.

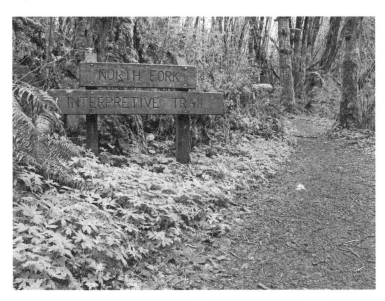

Trail 58. Clemens Park Loop

Length: 1-mile loop • **Elevation gain:** 15 feet
Difficulty: Easy • **Trail uses:** Foot, bike, horse
Trail surface: Packed earth
Seasonal closures: Closed to bikes and horses 10/31 to 4/15
Managing agency: Benton County

Start the loop from the parking lot, either next to the information kiosk by the bridge or from the corner by the restroom. Take an interpretive brochure for your walk and return it to the kiosk when you are done if you do not wish to keep it. The interpretive trail branches off from the path through the picnic area and follows along the river. One interpretive post focuses our attention on the streamside vegetation that helps stabilize the bank, provides shade for juvenile fish, and is an indicator of overall river health. Often blue herons and kingfishers can be observed along here, searching for their next meal. Another post is in an area representative of the forest understory with vine maple, salal, Oregon grape, and sword ferns up to 6 feet in diameter. Helping to nourish this rich understory are decaying nurse logs, lichens, and mosses that thrive in the cool temperaturess and plentiful moisture of this region. Up in the canopy, amongst the Douglas-firs, grand firs, and big-leaf maples, are some large Pacific yew trees. These

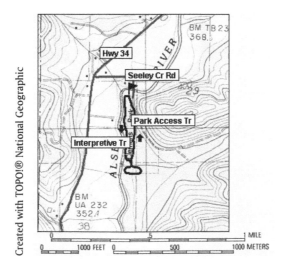

Created with TOPO!® National Geographic

trees were valued by the Native Americans for their hard, durable wood, and thus preferred for bows, salmon spears, paddles, and much more. Especially when the leaves have fallen, one can see licorice ferns growing high in the canopy on the branches of big-leaf maples. There is a well-constructed and well-placed salmon-watching deck and interpretive display done by an Eagle Scout. October is the best month to see salmon on their way to their ancestral spawning grounds.

The interpretive trail joins the park access trail. Turn right and continue downriver. Cross a bridge over Seeley Creek. Enhancement efforts have helped to make this stream a healthy habitat for salmon. The trail splits now and makes a loop. Heading to the right, there is a nice overlook of Seeley Creek, before continuing along the Alsea River. The trail then turns away from the river, looping through second-growth forest, before it arrives back at the bridge. To return to the parking lot, continue straight on the wide, graveled, and pleasant access trail. Notice the huge stumps from long-ago harvests that now look like vases holding bouquets of young forest plants. Enjoy this protected corridor; industrial forest lands are not far away.

Future Trails

In my citizen volunteer capacity with both Benton County Natural Areas and Parks Department and Corvallis Parks and Recreation Department, I know that additional trails are being planned for our area. Building a new trail is a long process. It begins with a vision. It then has to join the queue of projects also clamoring for attention and priority. Once there, it has to wait patiently, sometimes for a long time. Meanwhile, planning is being done and funding secured. Funding is quite often, at least in part, in the form of grants, and of course there are countless other projects all competing for these same monies. All the while, other projects beneficial to our community are being completed and the public land managing agencies are scrambling to maintain the extensive trail system we already have. This task, most assuredly, could not be accomplished without dedicated folks who volunteer their time, and their backs, for the simple reason that they love to have good trails to recreate on. Finally, our patiently waiting trail gets to the front of the line. Volunteer workers are recruited and trail building commences. Hours and hours of good old-fashioned labor goes into trail building. The result is a sturdy path that an infinite number of soles, paws, hooves, and knobby tires will tread upon for years to come.

There are several trail connections planned and/or under construction throughout the area. One of these is Marys River Natural Park. This is a 74-acre riparian wetland in the floodplain of the Marys River. It is situated east of Brooklane Drive off Hwy. 34/Philomath Blvd. Two phases of raised boardwalk have been constructed, including interpretive panels explaining the unique ecology of the area. The proposed next phase will take the boardwalk to the river and ultimately a pedestrian bridge is envisioned that will cross into Caldwell Open Space, another Corvallis Open Space property comprising 36 acres of lush riparian land. Additional trail extensions are planned. Natural habitat restoration is currently underway there.

Index

Y

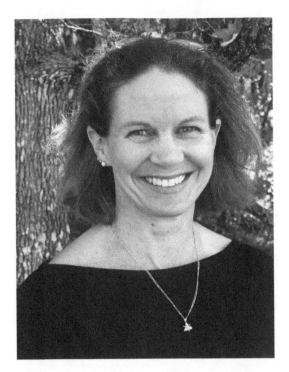

Margie Powell, a former U.S. Forest Service backcountry ranger, serves as trail work coordinator for the Marys Peak Group of the Sierra Club. A longtime supporter of parks and natural areas, she is a member of the City of Corvallis Open Space Commission and the Benton County Natural Areas and Parks Advisory Board. She has been living in Corvallis and recreating on local trails since 1993.

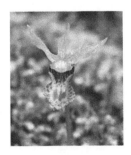